TITLE: AUTOIMMUNE PALEO DIET COOKBOOK

Healing Recipes for Wellness and Vitality

By

Nancy Bratton

Table of Contents

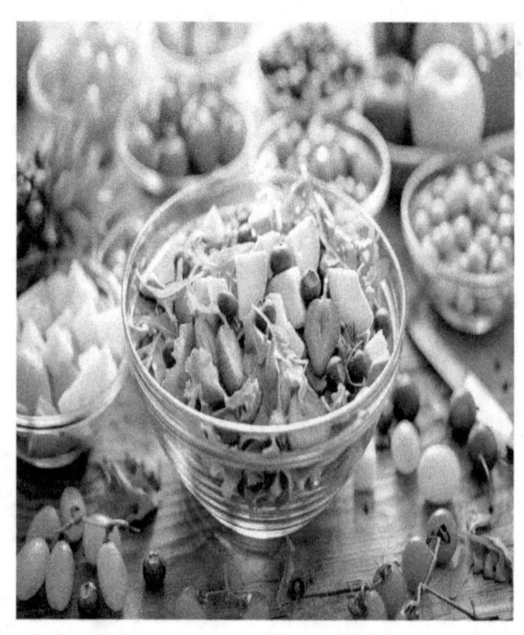

My Journey to the Autoimmune Paleo Diet

I used to be a food lover. Not just a casual enjoyer, but a fervent devotee. My world revolves around the next culinary adventure. From the bustling markets of Bangkok to the cozy bistros of Paris, I'd chased flavor with a zeal that bordered on obsession.

Then came the crash.

It started subtly: a persistent ache, a fatigue that no amount of coffee could conquer. I ignored it at first, attributing it to stress or overwork. But as the months turned into a year, these symptoms morphed into something more sinister. Joint pain, digestive distress, and a brain fog so thick, I felt like I was wading through molasses.

For years, I lived with a myriad of unexplained symptoms. Fatigue that left me drained by mid-afternoon, joint pain that made every movement a chore, and a foggy brain that often felt like I was wading through molasses. My once vibrant energy was replaced by a constant state of malaise. Numerous doctor visits yielded little more than vague diagnoses and prescriptions that offered minimal relief. I was at a crossroads, feeling like a stranger in my own body.

One evening, while scrolling through an online forum in desperation, I stumbled upon a thread about autoimmune diseases. As I read the stories of others who had experienced similar struggles, I saw a glimmer of my own life mirrored back at me. It was then that I first encountered the Autoimmune Paleo (AIP) diet. Skeptical but intrigued, I delved deeper into the research.

Making the decision to radically alter my diet wasn't easy. The AIP diet was strict, eliminating many foods I loved. But the more I read, the more I believed it could be the key to regaining my health. I decided to commit to a 30-day trial, fully aware that this journey would require dedication and resilience.

The first week was the hardest. I cleaned out my pantry, removing all non-compliant foods and stocked up on fresh vegetables, organic meats, and AIP-friendly snacks. Cooking became a daily ritual, a therapeutic process of transforming simple ingredients into nourishing meals. The initial cravings for sugar and grains were intense, but I found solace in the vibrant flavors of herbs and spices that brought my meals to life.

Embarking on the AIP was like trading my colorful palate for a monochrome existence. Gone were the days of rich curries, creamy pastas, and decadent desserts. In their place were bone broth, sweet potatoes, and a whole lot of experimentation. It was a journey fraught with frustration and loneliness. I missed the camaraderie of shared meals, the joy of discovering new tastes.

As the weeks passed, I began to notice subtle changes. The brain fog started to lift, and my energy levels stabilized. The joint pain that had been my constant companion for years began to subside. There were moments of doubt and temptation, especially during social gatherings where I had to explain my dietary choices. But the tangible improvements in my health were undeniable and kept me motivated.

One of the most profound moments came at the end of my first month on the AIP diet. I woke up one morning feeling genuinely refreshed for the first time in years. It was as if a heavy shroud had been lifted, revealing a glimpse of the vibrant life I had almost forgotten.

The AIP isn't just a diet; it's a lifestyle change. It's about listening to your body, honoring its needs, and finding joy in the process of healing. It's about discovering that true nourishment comes not just from what you eat, but from the overall well-being it brings. And while I may never be the food adventurer I once was, I've found a deeper appreciation for the flavors that truly nourish me, both physically and emotionally.

Connecting with others in the AIP community also played a crucial role in my journey. Sharing experiences, recipes, and encouragement created a support network that made the challenging days more bearable.

Today, as I look back at that lost and frightened woman, I see a survivor. A woman who, through adversity, found strength, resilience, and a renewed sense of purpose. And for that, I am eternally grateful.

Looking back, my journey to the Autoimmune Paleo diet has been transformative. It wasn't just about changing what I ate; it was about reclaiming control over my health and life. The AIP diet taught me to listen to my body, to nourish it with care, and to appreciate the small victories along the way.

Today, I continue to follow the AIP principles, albeit with a few personal modifications. My autoimmune symptoms are not entirely gone, but they are manageable, and I have regained a quality of life I once thought lost forever.

If you find yourself grappling with unexplained health issues, feeling lost in a sea of symptoms and diagnoses, consider exploring the AIP diet. It may be challenging, but the potential rewards are immense. My journey has shown me that with perseverance, support, and a willingness to change, it is possible to find healing and hope through the power of food.

The road to recovery is never linear, but every step forward is a step toward reclaiming your health and vitality. Embrace the journey, trust the process, and remember that you are not alone.

Introduction

Overview of Autoimmune Diseases

Autoimmune diseases occur when the body's immune system mistakenly attacks its own cells, leading to chronic inflammation and damage to various tissues and organs. More than 80 autoimmune disorders have been identified, including rheumatoid arthritis, lupus, multiple sclerosis, Hashimoto's thyroiditis, and psoriasis. Common symptoms can include fatigue, joint pain, muscle weakness, digestive issues, skin rashes, and cognitive difficulties. These symptoms can significantly affect an individual's quality of life and may vary in intensity and duration. The exact cause of autoimmune diseases is unknown, but genetic, environmental, and lifestyle factors are believed to contribute to their development. Diet plays a crucial role in managing autoimmune diseases by reducing inflammation, improving gut health, and supporting overall immune function.

The Paleo Diet

The Paleo diet, also known as the Paleolithic or caveman diet, is based on the types of foods presumed to have been eaten by early humans. This diet emphasizes whole, unprocessed foods such as vegetables, fruits, nuts, seeds, lean meats, and fish, while eliminating grains, legumes, dairy, and refined sugars. The rationale behind the Paleo diet is that modern agricultural practices have introduced foods that our bodies are not well adapted to, contributing to inflammation and autoimmune reactions. By focusing on nutrient-dense, anti-inflammatory foods, the Paleo diet aims to support the body's natural healing processes and reduce the burden on the immune system.

Why an Autoimmune Paleo Diet?
The Autoimmune Paleo (AIP) diet takes the principles of the Paleo diet a step further by specifically targeting foods that can trigger autoimmune responses. In addition to avoiding grains, legumes, dairy, and refined sugars, the AIP diet eliminates other potential irritants such as nightshades (e.g., tomatoes, peppers), nuts, seeds, and eggs. This approach helps identify food sensitivities and reduces inflammation, allowing the immune system to reset and function more effectively. By carefully reintroducing foods after an elimination period, individuals can determine which foods they can tolerate and which they should avoid to maintain optimal health.

The Paleo Autoimmune Protocol (AIP)
The Paleo Autoimmune Protocol (AIP) is an extension of the Paleo diet, specifically designed to help those with

autoimmune conditions. The AIP diet focuses on eliminating foods that are known to trigger inflammation and autoimmune reactions, allowing the body to heal and the immune system to reset. The protocol consists of two main phases:

1. Elimination Phase: During this phase, common inflammatory foods and potential irritants are removed from the diet. These include grains, legumes, dairy, refined sugars, processed foods, nightshades (such as tomatoes, peppers, and eggplants), nuts, seeds, eggs, and certain spices. The goal is to reduce overall inflammation and allow the gut to heal. This phase typically lasts for 30 to 90 days, depending on individual needs and symptom improvement.

2. Reintroduction Phase: Once symptoms have stabilized or improved, foods are slowly reintroduced one at a time to identify any potential triggers. This process helps individuals determine which foods they can tolerate and which they should avoid long-term. The reintroduction phase should be done carefully and methodically, with attention to any changes in symptoms.

Benefits of the AIP Diet

The AIP diet has been shown to provide several benefits for individuals with autoimmune conditions. These benefits are supported by scientific research and include:

1. Reduced Inflammation: The AIP diet eliminates common inflammatory foods and emphasizes nutrient-dense, anti-inflammatory foods. This reduction in inflammation can lead to a decrease in autoimmune symptoms and an overall improvement in health.

2. Improved Gut Health: Many autoimmune conditions are linked to poor gut health and increased intestinal permeability (leaky gut). The AIP diet includes foods that support gut healing, such as bone broth, fermented vegetables, and high-fiber vegetables. Improved gut health can enhance nutrient absorption and reduce autoimmune reactions.

3. Better Immune Function: By eliminating foods that can trigger immune responses, the AIP diet helps to balance and modulate the immune system. This can result in fewer flare-ups and a more stable, less reactive immune system.

4. Enhanced Nutrient Intake: The AIP diet focuses on whole, nutrient-dense foods that provide essential

vitamins, minerals, and antioxidants. These nutrients are crucial for supporting overall health and aiding in the repair and regeneration of tissues.

5. Personalized Dietary Insights: The reintroduction phase of the AIP diet allows individuals to identify specific food triggers and tailor their diet to their unique needs. This personalized approach can lead to long-term dietary habits that support optimal health and well-being.

Embark on this journey to reclaim your health and vitality with the Autoimmune Paleo Diet Cookbook. Let food be your medicine and discover the transformative power of eating in harmony with your body's needs.

By following the AIP diet, many individuals have experienced significant improvements in their autoimmune symptoms, energy levels, and overall quality of life. This cookbook is designed to guide you through the AIP journey with delicious, healing recipes and valuable insights into the science and benefits of the AIP diet. Embrace the power of food to transform your health and reclaim your vitality.

Chapter 1: Meal Planning and Preparation

Kitchen Essentials

AIP-Friendly Pantry Staples:
1. Proteins:
   - Grass-fed beef
   - Pasture-raised poultry
   - Wild-caught fish and seafood
   - Organ meats
   - Bone broth

2. Vegetables:
   - Leafy greens (spinach, kale, Swiss chard)
   - Cruciferous vegetables (broccoli, cauliflower, Brussels sprouts)
   - Root vegetables (sweet potatoes, carrots, beets)
   - Squash (butternut, acorn, zucchini)

3. Fruits:
   - Berries (blueberries, strawberries, raspberries)
   - Apples
   - Pears
   - Avocados

4. Fats:
   - Coconut oil

- Olive oil
- Avocado oil
- Animal fats (tallow, lard)

5. Herbs and Spices:
   - Basil
   - Thyme
   - Rosemary
   - Turmeric
   - Ginger

6. Fermented Foods:
   - Sauerkraut
   - Kimchi (without nightshades)
   - Coconut yogurt

7. Miscellaneous:
   - Coconut aminos
   - Apple cider vinegar
   - Arrowroot powder (for thickening)
   - Gelatin or collagen peptides

Kitchen Equipment:
1. Basic Tools:
   - Sharp chef's knife
   - Cutting board
   - Measuring cups and spoons
   - Mixing bowls

- Spatulas and wooden spoons

2. Cookware:
   - Cast iron skillet
   - Stainless steel pots and pans
   - Slow cooker or Instant Pot
   - Baking sheets
   - Glass storage containers

3. Appliances:
   - Blender or food processor
   - Immersion blender
   - Pressure cooker
   - Food dehydrator (optional)

Meal Planning Tips

1. Plan Ahead: Spend time each week planning your meals. Choose recipes that share common ingredients to minimize waste and streamline preparation.

2. Balance Your Plate: Ensure each meal includes a balance of protein, healthy fats, and a variety of vegetables. This helps maintain steady energy levels and provides a broad spectrum of nutrients.

3. Keep it Simple: Start with simple recipes, especially if you're new to the AIP diet. As you become more

comfortable, you can experiment with more complex dishes.

4. Use a Weekly Template: Create a template for your weekly meals (e.g., Meatless Mondays, Taco Tuesdays with lettuce wraps, etc.). This makes planning easier and adds variety to your diet.

5. Prep in Advance: Chop vegetables, marinate proteins, and prepare sauces or dressings in advance to save time during the week.

Batch Cooking

1. Double Recipes: When cooking, make double portions of recipes that freeze well, such as soups, stews, and casseroles. Freeze half for a future meal.

2. Cook Staples in Bulk: Prepare large batches of staple ingredients like roasted vegetables, grilled chicken, or steamed rice to use in multiple meals throughout the week.

3. Freezer-Friendly Meals: Stock your freezer with AIP-friendly meals that can be quickly reheated. Label containers with the date and contents for easy identification.

4. One-Pot Meals: Utilize one-pot or one-pan recipes to reduce cleanup time and make meal prep more efficient.

5. Set Aside Time: Dedicate a few hours each week, such as on weekends, for batch cooking and meal prep. This investment of time will pay off during busy weekdays when you can quickly assemble nutritious meals.

6. Use Your Tools: Make the most of your kitchen appliances. Use a slow cooker or Instant Pot for hands-off cooking, or a food processor to quickly chop vegetables and blend sauces.

By equipping your kitchen with the right tools and ingredients, planning your meals thoughtfully, and utilizing batch cooking techniques, you can create delicious, nutritious, and time-saving AIP meals that support your health and fit seamlessly into your lifestyle.

AIP Shopping Lists

Produce:
- Sweet potatoes
- Spinach
- Apples
- Mangos

- Asparagus
- Plantains
- Carrots
- Broccoli
- Zucchini
- Cauliflower
- Kale
- Cucumbers

Protein:
- Chicken breasts
- Ground sausage
- Salmon fillets
- Beef sirloin
- Turkey breast
- Lamb chops
- Pork tenderloin

Pantry Staples:
- Olive oil
- Coconut oil
- Coconut milk
- Bone broth
- Apple cider vinegar
- Honey or maple syrup
- Coconut aminos

Spices and Herbs:

- Cinnamon
- Garlic powder
- Ginger
- Basil
- Cilantro
- Dill
- Mint

Other:
- Coconut butter
- Coconut flour
- Almond flour
- Chia seeds
- Coconut yogurt

Produce:
- Large quantities of sweet potatoes, spinach, apples, mangos, asparagus, plantains, carrots, broccoli, zucchini, cauliflower, kale, cucumbers, and avocados

Protein:
- Large quantities of chicken breasts, ground sausage, salmon fillets, beef sirloin, turkey breast, lamb chops, pork tenderloin, and shrimp

Pantry Staples:

- Extra-large quantities of olive oil, coconut oil, coconut milk, bone broth, apple cider vinegar, honey or maple syrup, coconut aminos, and tahini

Spices and Herbs:
- Extra-large quantities of cinnamon, garlic powder, ginger, basil, cilantro, dill, and mint

Other:
- Extra-large quantities of coconut butter, coconut flour, almond flour, chia seeds, and coconut yogurt

Chapter 2: Breakfasts for Balanced Mornings

1.Gut-Healing Bone Broth Smoothie

Ingredients:
- 1 cup homemade bone broth
- 1 cup spinach leaves
- 1/2 avocado
- 1 small green apple, cored and chopped
- 1 tablespoon fresh lemon juice
- 1/2 teaspoon fresh ginger, grated
- Ice cubes (optional)

Instructions:
1. In a blender, combine bone broth, spinach, avocado, green apple, lemon juice, and ginger.
2. Blend until smooth, adding ice cubes if desired.
3. Pour into a glass and enjoy immediately.

Health Problems Addressed: Leaky gut syndrome, digestive issues

Health Benefits: Rich in collagen and amino acids for gut repair

Scientific Benefits: Collagen promotes gut health by supporting the lining of the digestive tract

"Since starting my day with this smoothie, I've noticed significantly less bloating and more consistent energy levels throughout the morning."

2.Anti-Inflammatory Sweet Potato Hash

Ingredients:
- 2 medium sweet potatoes, peeled and diced
- 1 tablespoon coconut oil
- 1 small onion, diced
- 1 bell pepper, diced (omit if nightshades are not tolerated)
- 1 teaspoon ground turmeric
- 1/2 teaspoon ground cumin
- Salt to taste
- Fresh parsley, chopped (for garnish)

Instructions:
1. In a large skillet, heat coconut oil over medium heat.
2. Add diced sweet potatoes and cook for 5-7 minutes, stirring occasionally.
3. Add onion and bell pepper, cooking until vegetables are tender.
4. Stir in turmeric, cumin, and salt. Cook for an additional 2-3 minutes.

5. Garnish with fresh parsley and serve.

Health Problems Addressed: Inflammation, joint pain

Health Benefits: High in antioxidants and anti-inflammatory compounds

Scientific Benefits: Sweet potatoes contain beta-carotene, which reduces inflammation

"This hash has become a staple in my breakfast routine. My joint pain has decreased, and I feel more mobile and energized."

3.Nutrient-Dense Green Smoothie Bowl

Ingredients:
- 1 cup coconut milk
- 1 cup spinach leaves
- 1/2 banana, frozen
- 1/2 avocado
- 1 tablespoon chia seeds
- 1 teaspoon spirulina powder (optional)
- Fresh berries, for topping
- Coconut flakes, for topping

Instructions:
1. In a blender, combine coconut milk, spinach, banana, avocado, chia seeds, and spirulina powder.
2. Blend until smooth and creamy.
3. Pour into a bowl and top with fresh berries and coconut flakes.

Health Problems Addressed: Fatigue, nutrient deficiencies

Health Benefits: Packed with vitamins, minerals, and healthy fats

Scientific Benefits: Greens like spinach and kale are rich in iron and magnesium, boosting energy levels

"Starting my day with this smoothie bowl has drastically improved my energy levels. I feel nourished and ready to take on the day."

4.Healing Chicken and Vegetable Soup (Breakfast Version)

Ingredients:
- 1 cup cooked, shredded chicken
- 1 cup bone broth
- 1/2 cup chopped carrots
- 1/2 cup chopped celery

- 1/2 cup chopped zucchini
- 1/2 teaspoon dried thyme
- 1/2 teaspoon dried oregano
- Salt to taste
- Fresh parsley, chopped (for garnish)

Instructions:
1. In a medium pot, bring bone broth to a simmer over medium heat.
2. Add carrots, celery, and zucchini. Cook until vegetables are tender.
3. Stir in shredded chicken, thyme, oregano, and salt. Cook for an additional 5 minutes.
4. Garnish with fresh parsley and serve warm.

Health Problems Addressed: Autoimmune flares, immune support

Health Benefits: Supports the immune system with vitamins and minerals

Scientific Benefits: Chicken broth is rich in vitamins and minerals that boost immune function

"Having this soup for breakfast has made a noticeable difference in how I feel throughout the day. My autoimmune flares are less frequent, and I feel more balanced."

5. Turmeric Cauliflower Scramble

Ingredients:
- 1 small head of cauliflower, grated (or 2 cups cauliflower rice)
- 1 tablespoon coconut oil
- 1/2 teaspoon ground turmeric
- 1/4 teaspoon ground black pepper
- 1/2 teaspoon sea salt
- 1/4 cup chopped green onions
- Fresh cilantro, for garnish

Instructions:
1. In a large skillet, heat coconut oil over medium heat.
2. Add grated cauliflower and cook for 5-7 minutes until tender.
3. Stir in turmeric, black pepper, and salt.
4. Add green onions and cook for another 2 minutes.
5. Garnish with fresh cilantro and serve warm.

Health Problems Addressed: Inflammation, digestive health

Health Benefits: Anti-inflammatory and high in fiber
Scientific Benefits: Turmeric's curcumin reduces inflammation; cauliflower is fiber-rich for digestive health

"This scramble is a flavorful and satisfying way to start my day. I've noticed less bloating and more regular digestion."

6. Coconut Yogurt Parfait

Ingredients:
- 1 cup coconut yogurt
- 1/2 cup mixed berries (blueberries, strawberries, raspberries)
- 2 tablespoons coconut flakes
- 1 tablespoon chia seeds

Instructions:
1. Layer coconut yogurt and mixed berries in a bowl or parfait glass.
2. Top with coconut flakes and chia seeds.
3. Enjoy immediately.

Health Problems Addressed: Gut health, nutrient deficiencies

Health Benefits: Probiotics for gut health, rich in vitamins and antioxidants

Scientific Benefits: Coconut yogurt contains probiotics; berries provide antioxidants and vitamins

"This parfait is delicious and keeps my gut health in check. I feel more energized and my digestion has improved."

7. Sweet Potato and Apple Hash

Ingredients:
- 2 medium sweet potatoes, diced
- 1 large apple, diced
- 1 tablespoon coconut oil
- 1 teaspoon ground cinnamon
- 1/2 teaspoon sea salt
- Fresh thyme, for garnish

Instructions:
1. In a large skillet, heat coconut oil over medium heat.
2. Add sweet potatoes and cook for 10 minutes, stirring occasionally.
3. Add apples, cinnamon, and salt. Cook for an additional 5 minutes.
4. Garnish with fresh thyme and serve warm.

Health Problems Addressed: Blood sugar regulation, inflammation

Health Benefits: Balanced blood sugar levels, anti-inflammatory properties

Scientific Benefits: Sweet potatoes have a low glycemic index; apples contain quercetin, an anti-inflammatory

"This hash is my go-to breakfast for staying full and balanced. My blood sugar levels have stabilized, and I feel great."

8. Avocado and Salmon Breakfast Salad

Ingredients:
- 2 cups mixed greens
- 1/2 avocado, sliced
- 1/2 cup cooked, flaked salmon
- 1 tablespoon olive oil
- 1 tablespoon fresh lemon juice
- Sea salt and black pepper to taste

Instructions:
1. In a large bowl, combine mixed greens, avocado, and salmon.
2. Drizzle with olive oil and lemon juice.
3. Season with salt and pepper, then toss to combine.
4. Serve immediately.

Health Problems Addressed: Heart health, brain function

Health Benefits: Rich in omega-3 fatty acids and antioxidants

Scientific Benefits: Salmon provides omega-3s for heart and brain health; avocados offer healthy fats and vitamins

"This salad is a refreshing and filling breakfast. My heart health has improved, and I feel more mentally sharp."

9. Apple-Cinnamon Breakfast Porridge

Ingredients:
- 1/2 cup unsweetened applesauce
- 1/2 cup coconut milk
- 1/4 cup shredded coconut
- 1/2 teaspoon ground cinnamon
- 1 tablespoon chia seeds
- Fresh apple slices, for topping

Instructions:
1. In a small saucepan, combine applesauce, coconut milk, shredded coconut, cinnamon, and chia seeds.
2. Cook over medium heat, stirring frequently, until thickened (about 5 minutes).
3. Pour into a bowl and top with fresh apple slices.
4. Serve warm.

Health Problems Addressed: Digestive health, inflammation

Health Benefits: High in fiber and anti-inflammatory compounds

Scientific Benefits: Applesauce and chia seeds provide fiber; cinnamon has anti-inflammatory properties

"This porridge is comforting and helps with my digestion. I've noticed less inflammation and more regular bowel movements."

10. Bacon and Butternut Squash Breakfast Bake

Ingredients:
- 4 slices of nitrate-free bacon, chopped
- 2 cups butternut squash, peeled and diced
- 1 small onion, diced
- 1 tablespoon coconut oil
- 1 teaspoon dried sage
- 1/2 teaspoon sea salt
- Fresh parsley, for garnish

Instructions:
1. Preheat the oven to 375°F (190°C).
2. In a large skillet, cook bacon over medium heat until crispy. Remove and set aside.

3. In the same skillet, add coconut oil, butternut squash, and onion. Cook for 10 minutes until tender.
4. Stir in sage and salt, then transfer to a baking dish.
5. Top with cooked bacon and bake for 20 minutes.
6. Garnish with fresh parsley and serve warm.

Health Problems Addressed: Blood sugar regulation, inflammation

Health Benefits: Balanced blood sugar levels, anti-inflammatory properties

Scientific Benefits: Butternut squash has a low glycemic index; bacon (when nitrate-free) can be part of a balanced diet

"This bake is hearty and satisfying. It keeps my blood sugar stable and reduces inflammation."

11. Carrot and Zucchini Breakfast Muffins

Ingredients:
- 1 cup grated carrots
- 1 cup grated zucchini
- 1/4 cup coconut flour
- 1/4 cup coconut oil, melted
- 1 tablespoon ground flaxseed
- 1/2 teaspoon baking soda

- 1/2 teaspoon ground cinnamon
- 1/4 teaspoon sea salt

Instructions:
1. Preheat the oven to 350°F (175°C).
2. In a large bowl, combine all ingredients and mix well.
3. Divide the batter into a greased muffin tin.
4. Bake for 20-25 minutes, or until a toothpick inserted comes out clean.
5. Let cool before serving.

Health Problems Addressed: Nutrient deficiencies, inflammation

Health Benefits: High in vitamins and anti-inflammatory compounds

Scientific Benefits: Carrots and zucchini are rich in vitamins A and C; coconut flour provides fiber

"These muffins are a perfect grab-and-go breakfast. They're delicious and keep me full and energized."

12. Berry-Coconut Chia Pudding

Ingredients:
- 1 cup coconut milk
- 1/4 cup chia seeds

- 1/2 cup mixed berries
- 1 tablespoon shredded coconut

Instructions:
1. In a bowl, mix coconut milk and chia seeds. Let sit for 10 minutes, then stir again.
2. Cover and refrigerate overnight.
3. In the morning, top with mixed berries and shredded coconut.
4. Serve chilled.

Health Problems Addressed: Gut health, nutrient deficiencies

Health Benefits: High in fiber, antioxidants, and healthy fats

Scientific Benefits: Chia seeds provide fiber and omega-3s; berries are rich in antioxidants

"This chia pudding is a refreshing and nutritious way to start my day. It keeps my digestion regular and my energy levels high."

13. Kale and Sweet Potato Breakfast Skillet

Ingredients:
- 1 tablespoon coconut oil

- 2 cups chopped kale
- 1 medium sweet potato, diced
- 1 small onion, diced
- 1/2 teaspoon ground turmeric
- Sea salt and black pepper to taste

Instructions:
1. In a large skillet, heat coconut oil over medium heat.
2. Add sweet potato and onion, cooking for 10 minutes until tender.
3. Stir in kale, turmeric, salt, and pepper. Cook for another 5 minutes until kale is wilted.
4. Serve warm.

Health Problems Addressed: Inflammation, nutrient deficiencies

Health Benefits: High in vitamins, minerals, and anti-inflammatory compounds

Scientific Benefits: Kale provides vitamins K and C; sweet potatoes contain beta-carotene

"This skillet is a powerhouse of nutrients. It's delicious and makes me feel nourished and energized."

14. Cinnamon-Apple Breakfast Sausage Patties

Ingredients:
- 1 pound ground pork
- 1 apple, peeled and grated
- 1 teaspoon ground cinnamon
- 1/2 teaspoon sea salt
- 1/4 teaspoon ground black pepper
- Coconut oil for frying

Instructions:
1. In a bowl, combine ground pork, grated apple, cinnamon, salt, and pepper.
2. Form into small patties.
3. In a skillet, heat coconut oil over medium heat.
4. Cook patties for 5-7 minutes on each side until fully cooked.
5. Serve warm.

Health Problems Addressed: Inflammation, nutrient deficiencies

Health Benefits: High in protein and anti-inflammatory compounds

Scientific Benefits: Pork provides protein and essential nutrients; apples offer antioxidants and fiber

"These sausage patties are a hit in my household. They're flavorful and keep us satisfied all morning."

15. Banana-Coconut Pancakes

Ingredients:
- 2 ripe bananas, mashed
- 2 eggs
- 1/4 cup coconut flour
- 1/4 cup coconut milk
- 1/2 teaspoon baking soda
- Coconut oil for cooking

Instructions:
1. In a bowl, combine mashed bananas, eggs, coconut flour, coconut milk, and baking soda.
2. Heat coconut oil in a skillet over medium heat.
3. Pour batter into the skillet, forming small pancakes.
4. Cook for 2-3 minutes on each side until golden brown.
5. Serve warm with fresh berries or coconut yogurt.

Health Problems Addressed: Blood sugar regulation, nutrient deficiencies

Health Benefits: Balanced blood sugar levels, high in vitamins and healthy fats

Scientific Benefits: Bananas provide potassium; coconut flour and milk are rich in healthy fats and fiber

"These pancakes are a weekend favorite. They're delicious and don't spike my blood sugar like regular pancakes."

16. Spinach and Avocado Breakfast Salad

Ingredients:
- 2 cups baby spinach leaves
- 1/2 avocado, sliced
- 1/2 cup cherry tomatoes, halved (omit if nightshades are not tolerated)
- 1 tablespoon olive oil
- 1 tablespoon lemon juice
- Sea salt and black pepper to taste

Instructions:
1. In a large bowl, combine spinach, avocado, and cherry tomatoes.
2. Drizzle with olive oil and lemon juice.
3. Season with salt and pepper, then toss to combine.
4. Serve immediately.

Health Problems Addressed: Heart health, nutrient deficiencies

Health Benefits: Rich in vitamins, minerals, and healthy fats

Scientific Benefits: Spinach provides iron and magnesium; avocado offers healthy fats and vitamins

"This salad is light yet satisfying. It's perfect for a healthy start to my day and keeps me feeling full and balanced."

17. Butternut Squash and Apple Breakfast Soup

Ingredients:
- 1 tablespoon coconut oil
- 1 small onion, diced
- 1 medium butternut squash, peeled and cubed
- 1 large apple, peeled and chopped
- 4 cups bone broth
- 1 teaspoon ground cinnamon
- 1/2 teaspoon sea salt
- Fresh thyme, for garnish

Instructions:
1. In a large pot, heat coconut oil over medium heat.
2. Add onion and cook until translucent.
3. Add butternut squash, apple, bone broth, cinnamon, and salt.
4. Bring to a boil, then reduce heat and simmer for 20 minutes until squash is tender.
5. Use an immersion blender to puree the soup until smooth.

6. Garnish with fresh thyme and serve warm.

Health Problems Addressed: Inflammation, digestive health

Health Benefits: High in vitamins, anti-inflammatory compounds, and fiber

Scientific Benefits: Butternut squash and apples provide vitamins A and C; bone broth supports gut health

"This soup is comforting and nourishing. It's my go-to breakfast during colder months, and it helps with my digestion."

18. Coconut Flour Waffles

Ingredients:
- 1/2 cup coconut flour
- 4 eggs
- 1/4 cup coconut milk
- 1/4 cup melted coconut oil
- 1/2 teaspoon baking soda
- 1/2 teaspoon sea salt
- Coconut oil for greasing the waffle iron

Instructions:
1. Preheat the waffle iron and grease with coconut oil.

2. In a bowl, mix coconut flour, eggs, coconut milk, melted coconut oil, baking soda, and salt until smooth.
3. Pour batter into the waffle iron and cook according to the manufacturer's instructions.
4. Serve warm with fresh berries or coconut yogurt.

Health Problems Addressed: Blood sugar regulation, nutrient deficiencies

Health Benefits: Balanced blood sugar levels, high in vitamins and healthy fats

Scientific Benefits: Coconut flour is low in carbs and high in fiber; eggs provide protein and essential nutrients

"These waffles are a weekend treat. They're light and fluffy, and keep me satisfied without a sugar crash."

19. AIP-Friendly Breakfast Burrito

Ingredients:
- 2 large collard green leaves, stems removed
- 1/2 cup cooked ground turkey
- 1/4 cup diced sweet potato, cooked
- 1/4 avocado, sliced
- 1 tablespoon coconut aminos
- 1 teaspoon fresh lime juice
- Sea salt and black pepper to taste

Instructions:
1. In a skillet, heat ground turkey and diced sweet potato until warmed through.
2. Season with coconut aminos, lime juice, salt, and pepper.
3. Place collard green leaves on a flat surface and layer with turkey mixture and avocado slices.
4. Roll up the leaves to form a burrito.
5. Serve immediately.

Health Problems Addressed: Inflammation, nutrient deficiencies

Health Benefits: High in protein, vitamins, and healthy fats

Scientific Benefits: Collard greens are rich in vitamins A, C, and K; avocado provides healthy fats

"This breakfast burrito is a great way to start my day. It's filling and packed with nutrients, helping me stay energized."

20. Cauliflower and Apple Breakfast Bowl

Ingredients:
- 2 cups cauliflower rice

- 1 large apple, peeled and chopped
- 1/2 cup coconut milk
- 1 tablespoon coconut oil
- 1 teaspoon ground cinnamon
- 1/4 teaspoon sea salt
- Fresh berries, for topping

Instructions:
1. In a large skillet, heat coconut oil over medium heat.
2. Add cauliflower rice and cook for 5 minutes until tender.
3. Stir in chopped apple, coconut milk, cinnamon, and salt.
4. Cook for an additional 5 minutes until the apple is tender and the mixture is heated through.
5. Serve warm, topped with fresh berries.

Health Problems Addressed: Blood sugar regulation, nutrient deficiencies

Health Benefits: Balanced blood sugar levels, high in fiber and vitamins

Scientific Benefits: Cauliflower provides fiber; apples offer antioxidants and vitamins

"This breakfast bowl is hearty and nutritious. It keeps my blood sugar stable and gives me lasting energy."

21. Beet and Avocado Smoothie

Ingredients:
- 1 small beet, peeled and chopped
- 1/2 avocado
- 1 cup coconut milk
- 1 small banana, frozen
- 1 tablespoon chia seeds
- 1 teaspoon fresh lemon juice

Instructions:
1. In a blender, combine beet, avocado, coconut milk, banana, chia seeds, and lemon juice.
2. Blend until smooth.
3. Pour into a glass and enjoy immediately.

Health Problems Addressed: Detoxification, nutrient deficiencies

Health Benefits: Rich in vitamins, minerals, and antioxidants

Scientific Benefits: Beets are high in folate and manganese; avocado provides healthy fats and potassium

"This smoothie is both vibrant and refreshing. It helps detoxify my body and provides sustained energy."

22. Pumpkin-Spice Breakfast Pudding

Ingredients:
- 1 cup pumpkin puree
- 1/2 cup coconut milk
- 1/4 cup chia seeds
- 1 tablespoon maple syrup (optional)
- 1 teaspoon pumpkin spice blend
- Fresh berries, for topping

Instructions:
1. In a bowl, mix pumpkin puree, coconut milk, chia seeds, maple syrup, and pumpkin spice blend.
2. Let sit for 10 minutes, then stir again.
3. Cover and refrigerate overnight.
4. Top with fresh berries before serving.

Health Problems Addressed: Inflammation, digestive health

Health Benefits: High in fiber, vitamins, and antioxidants

Scientific Benefits: Pumpkin is rich in beta-carotene; chia seeds provide omega-3 fatty acids

"This pudding is a delicious way to enjoy pumpkin year-round. It keeps me full and my digestion regular."

23. Sage and Apple Breakfast Sausages

Ingredients:
- 1 pound ground turkey
- 1 apple, peeled and grated
- 1 teaspoon dried sage
- 1/2 teaspoon sea salt
- 1/4 teaspoon ground black pepper
- Coconut oil for frying

Instructions:
1. In a bowl, combine ground turkey, grated apple, sage, salt, and pepper.
2. Form into small patties.
3. In a skillet, heat coconut oil over medium heat.
4. Cook patties for 5-7 minutes on each side until fully cooked.
5. Serve warm.

Health Problems Addressed: Inflammation, nutrient deficiencies

Health Benefits: High in protein and anti-inflammatory compounds

Scientific Benefits: Turkey provides lean protein; sage has anti-inflammatory properties

"These sausages are a great addition to my breakfast routine. They're flavorful and help with my inflammation."

24. AIP-Friendly Breakfast Tacos

Ingredients:
- 2 large collard green leaves, stems removed
- 1/2 cup cooked ground beef
- 1/4 cup diced sweet potato, cooked
- 1/4 avocado, sliced
- 1 tablespoon coconut aminos
- 1 teaspoon fresh lime juice
- Sea salt and black pepper to taste

Instructions:
1. In a skillet, heat ground beef and diced sweet potato until warmed through.
2. Season with coconut aminos, lime juice, salt, and pepper.
3. Place collard green leaves on a flat surface and layer with beef mixture and avocado slices.
4. Roll up the leaves to form tacos.
5. Serve immediately.

Health Problems Addressed: Inflammation, nutrient deficiencies

Health Benefits: High in protein, vitamins, and healthy fats

Scientific Benefits: Collard greens are rich in vitamins A, C, and K; avocado provides healthy fats

"These breakfast tacos are both nutritious and satisfying. They help me stay energized and reduce inflammation."

25. Blueberry-Coconut Breakfast Bars

Ingredients:
- 1 cup shredded coconut
- 1/2 cup coconut flour
- 1/2 cup coconut oil, melted
- 1/4 cup honey
- 1 cup fresh blueberries

Instructions:
1. Preheat the oven to 350°F (175°C).
2. In a bowl, mix shredded coconut, coconut flour, coconut oil, and honey.
3. Fold in fresh blueberries.
4. Press the mixture into a greased baking dish.
5. Bake for 20-25 minutes until golden brown.
6. Let cool before cutting into bars.

Health Problems Addressed: Inflammation, blood sugar regulation

Health Benefits: High in healthy fats and antioxidants

Scientific Benefits: Blueberries are rich in antioxidants; coconut flour is low in carbs and high in fiber

"These bars are a convenient and tasty breakfast option. They keep me full and my blood sugar stable."

26. Zucchini and Herb Breakfast Frittata

Ingredients:
- 1 tablespoon coconut oil
- 1 small onion, diced
- 1 zucchini, grated
- 1/4 cup chopped fresh herbs (parsley, basil, dill)
- 4 eggs
- Sea salt and black pepper to taste

Instructions:
1. Preheat the oven to 375°F (190°C).
2. In a skillet, heat coconut oil over medium heat. Add onion and cook until translucent.
3. Add grated zucchini and cook for another 5 minutes.
4. In a bowl, whisk eggs, fresh herbs, salt, and pepper.

5. Pour egg mixture into the skillet and cook for 2 minutes until edges start to set.

6. Transfer the skillet to the oven and bake for 15-20 minutes until fully set.

7. Let cool slightly before slicing and serving.

Health Problems Addressed: Inflammation, nutrient deficiencies

Health Benefits: High in protein, vitamins, and anti-inflammatory compounds

Scientific Benefits: Zucchini is rich in vitamins A and C; eggs provide protein and essential nutrients

"This frittata is a great way to start my day. It's delicious and keeps me full and satisfied."

27. Carrot-Apple Breakfast Muffins

Ingredients:
- 1 cup grated carrots
- 1 apple, peeled and grated
- 1/4 cup coconut flour
- 1/4 cup coconut oil, melted
- 1 tablespoon ground flaxseed
- 1/2 teaspoon baking soda
- 1/2 teaspoon ground cinnamon

- 1/4 teaspoon sea salt

Instructions:
1. Preheat the oven to 350°F (175°C).
2. In a large bowl, combine all ingredients and mix well.
3. Divide the batter into a greased muffin tin.
4. Bake for 20-25 minutes, or until a toothpick inserted comes out clean.
5. Let cool before serving.

Health Problems Addressed: Nutrient deficiencies, inflammation

Health Benefits: High in vitamins and anti-inflammatory compounds

Scientific Benefits: Carrots and apples are rich in vitamins A and C; coconut flour provides fiber

"These muffins are a perfect grab-and-go breakfast. They're delicious and keep me full and energized."

28. Ginger-Turmeric Smoothie

Ingredients:
- 1 cup coconut milk
- 1 small banana, frozen
- 1/2 teaspoon fresh ginger, grated

- 1/2 teaspoon ground turmeric
- 1 tablespoon chia seeds
- 1 teaspoon fresh lemon juice

Instructions:

1. In a blender, combine coconut milk, banana, ginger, turmeric, chia seeds, and lemon juice.
2. Blend until smooth.
3. Pour into a glass and enjoy immediately.

Health Problems Addressed: Inflammation, digestive health

Health Benefits: Anti-inflammatory and rich in antioxidants

Scientific Benefits: Turmeric and ginger have strong anti-inflammatory properties; chia seeds provide omega-3 fatty acids

"This smoothie is both flavorful and healing. It helps with my digestion and reduces inflammation."

29. Sweet Potato and Avocado Breakfast Toast

Ingredients:

- 1 large sweet potato, sliced into 1/4-inch thick slices
- 1/2 avocado, mashed

- 1 tablespoon fresh lemon juice
- Sea salt and black pepper to taste
- Fresh cilantro, for garnish

Instructions:
1. Preheat the oven to 375°F (190°C).
2. Arrange sweet potato slices on a baking sheet and bake for 15-20 minutes until tender.
3. In a bowl, combine mashed avocado, lemon juice, salt, and pepper.
4. Spread avocado mixture on baked sweet potato slices.
5. Garnish with fresh cilantro and serve warm.

Health Problems Addressed: Inflammation, blood sugar regulation

Health Benefits: Balanced blood sugar levels and anti-inflammatory properties

Scientific Benefits: Sweet potatoes have a low glycemic index; avocado provides healthy fats

"This breakfast toast is delicious and satisfying. It keeps my blood sugar stable and my energy levels high."

30. Cucumber and Dill Breakfast Salad

Ingredients:

- 2 cups chopped cucumber
- 1/4 cup chopped fresh dill
- 1/4 cup coconut yogurt
- 1 tablespoon fresh lemon juice
- Sea salt and black pepper to taste

Instructions:
1. In a large bowl, combine chopped cucumber, fresh dill, coconut yogurt, lemon juice, salt, and pepper.
2. Toss to combine.
3. Serve immediately.

Health Problems Addressed: Inflammation, digestive health

Health Benefits: Hydrating and anti-inflammatory

Scientific Benefits: Cucumbers are hydrating and rich in antioxidants; dill has antimicrobial properties

"This salad is refreshing and light. It's perfect for a healthy start to my day and helps with my digestion."

31. Apple and Cinnamon Breakfast Bowl

Ingredients:
- 1 large apple, peeled and chopped
- 1/2 cup coconut milk

- 1 tablespoon chia seeds
- 1 teaspoon ground cinnamon
- 1 tablespoon honey (optional)
- Fresh berries, for topping

Instructions:
1. In a bowl, mix chopped apple, coconut milk, chia seeds, cinnamon, and honey.
2. Let sit for 10 minutes to allow chia seeds to thicken.
3. Serve topped with fresh berries.

Health Problems Addressed: Blood sugar regulation, inflammation

Health Benefits: Balanced blood sugar levels and anti-inflammatory properties

Scientific Benefits: Apples are rich in antioxidants; chia seeds provide omega-3 fatty acids

"This breakfast bowl is both tasty and nutritious. It keeps my blood sugar stable and helps with inflammation."

32. Parsnip and Apple Hash

Ingredients:
- 1 tablespoon coconut oil
- 1 small onion, diced

- 2 parsnips, peeled and grated
- 1 apple, peeled and chopped
- 1 teaspoon fresh thyme
- Sea salt and black pepper to taste

Instructions:

1. In a skillet, heat coconut oil over medium heat. Add onion and cook until translucent.
2. Add grated parsnips and chopped apple. Cook for 10 minutes until tender.
3. Season with fresh thyme, salt, and pepper.
4. Serve warm.

Health Problems Addressed: Nutrient deficiencies, inflammation

Health Benefits: High in fiber and vitamins

Scientific Benefits: Parsnips are rich in fiber and vitamins; apples provide antioxidants

"This hash is a hearty and nutritious breakfast option. It keeps me full and helps with inflammation."

33. Kale and Avocado Smoothie

Ingredients:

- 1 cup kale leaves, chopped

- 1/2 avocado
- 1 small banana, frozen
- 1 cup coconut milk
- 1 tablespoon chia seeds
- 1 teaspoon fresh lemon juice

Instructions:
1. In a blender, combine kale, avocado, banana, coconut milk, chia seeds, and lemon juice.
2. Blend until smooth.
3. Pour into a glass and enjoy immediately.

Health Problems Addressed: Inflammation, nutrient deficiencies

Health Benefits: Anti-inflammatory and rich in vitamins and minerals

Scientific Benefits: Kale is rich in vitamins K, A, and C; avocado provides healthy fats

"This smoothie is a powerhouse of nutrients. It helps reduce inflammation and gives me lasting energy."

34. Turkey and Spinach Breakfast Scramble

Ingredients:
- 1 tablespoon coconut oil

- 1 small onion, diced
- 1 cup baby spinach leaves
- 1/2 cup cooked ground turkey
- 4 eggs
- Sea salt and black pepper to taste

Instructions:

1. In a skillet, heat coconut oil over medium heat. Add onion and cook until translucent.
2. Add spinach and cook until wilted.
3. Add ground turkey and cook until warmed through.
4. In a bowl, whisk eggs, salt, and pepper. Pour into the skillet.
5. Cook, stirring frequently, until eggs are fully cooked.
6. Serve warm.

Health Problems Addressed: Inflammation, nutrient deficiencies

Health Benefits: High in protein and vitamins

Scientific Benefits: Spinach is rich in iron and magnesium; turkey provides lean protein

"This scramble is a perfect way to start my day. It's filling and packed with nutrients."

35. Carrot and Zucchini Breakfast Muffins

Ingredients:
- 1 cup grated carrots
- 1 cup grated zucchini
- 1/4 cup coconut flour
- 1/4 cup coconut oil, melted
- 1 tablespoon ground flaxseed
- 1/2 teaspoon baking soda
- 1/2 teaspoon ground cinnamon
- 1/4 teaspoon sea salt

Instructions:
1. Preheat the oven to 350°F (175°C).
2. In a large bowl, combine all ingredients and mix well.
3. Divide the batter into a greased muffin tin.
4. Bake for 20-25 minutes, or until a toothpick inserted comes out clean.
5. Let cool before serving.

Health Problems Addressed: Nutrient deficiencies, inflammation

Health Benefits: High in vitamins and anti-inflammatory compounds

Scientific Benefits: Carrots and zucchini are rich in vitamins A and C; coconut flour provides fiber

"These muffins are a perfect grab-and-go breakfast. They're delicious and keep me full and energized."

36. Berry and Coconut Breakfast Parfait

Ingredients:
- 1 cup coconut yogurt
- 1/2 cup fresh berries
- 1 tablespoon chia seeds
- 1 tablespoon unsweetened shredded coconut

Instructions:
1. In a glass, layer coconut yogurt, fresh berries, chia seeds, and shredded coconut.
2. Repeat layers as desired.
3. Serve immediately.

Health Problems Addressed: Inflammation, digestive health

Health Benefits: High in probiotics, antioxidants, and healthy fats

Scientific Benefits: Berries are rich in antioxidants; coconut yogurt provides probiotics

"This parfait is both delicious and refreshing. It helps with my digestion and keeps me satisfied."

37. Sweet Potato and Apple Breakfast Bake

Ingredients:
- 1 large sweet potato, peeled and cubed
- 1 apple, peeled and chopped
- 1 tablespoon coconut oil, melted
- 1 teaspoon ground cinnamon
- 1/4 teaspoon sea salt
- Fresh thyme, for garnish

Instructions:
1. Preheat the oven to 375°F (190°C).
2. In a bowl, mix sweet potato, apple, coconut oil, cinnamon, and salt.
3. Spread mixture in a greased baking dish.
4. Bake for 25-30 minutes until the sweet potatoes are tender.
5. Garnish with fresh thyme and serve warm.

Health Problems Addressed: Inflammation, blood sugar regulation

Health Benefits: Balanced blood sugar levels and anti-inflammatory properties

Scientific Benefits: Sweet potatoes have a low glycemic index; apples provide antioxidants

"This breakfast bake is comforting and nutritious. It keeps my blood sugar stable and my energy levels high."

38. Avocado and Egg Breakfast Salad

Ingredients:
- 2 cups mixed greens
- 1/2 avocado, sliced
- 2 hard-boiled eggs, sliced
- 1 tablespoon olive oil
- 1 tablespoon fresh lemon juice
- Sea salt and black pepper to taste

Instructions:
1. In a large bowl, combine mixed greens, avocado, and hard-boiled eggs.
2. Drizzle with olive oil and lemon juice.
3. Season with salt and pepper, then toss to combine.
4. Serve immediately.

Health Problems Addressed: Inflammation, nutrient deficiencies

Health Benefits: High in protein, vitamins, and healthy fats

Scientific Benefits: Mixed greens are rich in vitamins and minerals; eggs provide protein and essential nutrients

"This salad is light yet filling. It's perfect for a healthy start to my day and helps with inflammation."

39. Apple-Cinnamon Overnight "Oats"

Ingredients:
- 1/2 cup unsweetened applesauce
- 1/4 cup coconut milk
- 1/4 cup chia seeds
- 1 teaspoon ground cinnamon
- 1 tablespoon honey (optional)
- Fresh berries, for topping

Instructions:
1. In a bowl, mix applesauce, coconut milk, chia seeds, cinnamon, and honey.
2. Cover and refrigerate overnight.
3. Serve topped with fresh berries.

Health Problems Addressed: Inflammation, blood sugar regulation

Health Benefits: Balanced blood sugar levels and anti-inflammatory properties

Scientific Benefits: Applesauce is rich in antioxidants; chia seeds provide omega-3 fatty acids

"These overnight 'oats' are a convenient and tasty breakfast. They keep my blood sugar stable and my energy levels high."

40. Turkey and Sweet Potato Breakfast Skillet

Ingredients:
- 1 tablespoon coconut oil
- 1 small onion, diced
- 1 cup diced sweet potato
- 1/2 cup cooked ground turkey
- 2 eggs
- Sea salt and black pepper to taste
- Fresh parsley, for garnish

Instructions:
1. In a skillet, heat coconut oil over medium heat. Add onion and cook until translucent.
2. Add diced sweet potato and cook for 10 minutes until tender.
3. Add ground turkey and cook until warmed through.
4. Make two wells in the skillet and crack an egg into each.
5. Cover and cook until eggs are set.

6. Season with salt and pepper and garnish with fresh parsley before serving.

Health Problems Addressed: Inflammation, nutrient deficiencies

Health Benefits: High in protein, vitamins, and anti-inflammatory compounds

Scientific Benefits: Sweet potatoes have a low glycemic index; turkey provides lean protein

"This skillet breakfast is hearty and satisfying. It keeps me full and my blood sugar stable."

41. Spaghetti Squash and Avocado Breakfast Bowl

Ingredients:
- 1 small spaghetti squash, cooked and shredded
- 1/2 avocado, sliced
- 1/4 cup cherry tomatoes, halved
- 1 tablespoon fresh lime juice
- Sea salt and black pepper to taste
- Fresh cilantro, for garnish

Instructions:
1. In a bowl, combine cooked spaghetti squash, avocado, and cherry tomatoes.

2. Drizzle with fresh lime juice and season with salt and pepper.
3. Toss gently to combine.
4. Garnish with fresh cilantro and serve immediately.

Health Problems Addressed: Inflammation, nutrient deficiencies

Health Benefits: High in vitamins and healthy fats

Scientific Benefits: Spaghetti squash is low in calories and high in fiber; avocado provides healthy fats

"This bowl is light, fresh, and filling. It's a perfect start to my day and keeps me satisfied."

42. Coconut and Blueberry Chia Pudding

Ingredients:
- 1 cup coconut milk
- 1/4 cup chia seeds
- 1 tablespoon honey (optional)
- 1/2 cup fresh blueberries

Instructions:
1. In a bowl, mix coconut milk, chia seeds, and honey.
2. Let sit for 10 minutes, then stir again.
3. Cover and refrigerate overnight.

4. Top with fresh blueberries before serving.

Health Problems Addressed: Inflammation, digestive health

Health Benefits: High in omega-3 fatty acids and antioxidants

Scientific Benefits: Chia seeds provide omega-3s; blueberries are rich in antioxidants

"This pudding is a delicious and easy breakfast. It helps with my digestion and reduces inflammation."

43. Butternut Squash and Sage Breakfast Hash

Ingredients:
- 1 tablespoon coconut oil
- 1 small onion, diced
- 1 cup butternut squash, peeled and cubed
- 1/2 teaspoon dried sage
- Sea salt and black pepper to taste
- Fresh parsley, for garnish

Instructions:
1. In a skillet, heat coconut oil over medium heat. Add onion and cook until translucent.

2. Add butternut squash and cook for 10-15 minutes until tender.

3. Season with dried sage, salt, and pepper.

4. Garnish with fresh parsley and serve warm.

Health Problems Addressed: Inflammation, nutrient deficiencies

Health Benefits: High in vitamins and anti-inflammatory compounds

Scientific Benefits: Butternut squash is rich in vitamins A and C; sage has anti-inflammatory properties

"This hash is warm, comforting, and packed with nutrients. It keeps me full and energized."

44. Apple and Walnut Breakfast Salad

Ingredients:
- 2 cups mixed greens
- 1 apple, sliced
- 1/4 cup chopped walnuts
- 1 tablespoon olive oil
- 1 tablespoon fresh lemon juice
- Sea salt and black pepper to taste

Instructions:

1. In a large bowl, combine mixed greens, apple slices,
and chopped walnuts.
2. Drizzle with olive oil and lemon juice.
3. Season with salt and pepper, then toss to combine.
4. Serve immediately.

Health Problems Addressed: Inflammation, nutrient
deficiencies

Health Benefits: High in vitamins, healthy fats, and
antioxidants

Scientific Benefits: Apples are rich in antioxidants;
walnuts provide omega-3 fatty acids

"This salad is refreshing and delicious. It's a great way to
start my day with a boost of nutrients."

45. Sweet Potato and Kale Breakfast Bowl

Ingredients:
- 1 tablespoon coconut oil
- 1 small sweet potato, peeled and cubed
- 1 cup kale leaves, chopped
- 1/4 cup cooked ground turkey
- 1 tablespoon coconut aminos
- Sea salt and black pepper to taste

Instructions:
1. In a skillet, heat coconut oil over medium heat. Add sweet potato and cook for 10-15 minutes until tender.
2. Add chopped kale and cook until wilted.
3. Add cooked ground turkey and season with coconut aminos, salt, and pepper.
4. Serve warm.

Health Problems Addressed: Inflammation, nutrient deficiencies

Health Benefits: High in protein, vitamins, and anti-inflammatory compounds

Scientific Benefits: Sweet potatoes are rich in vitamins A and C; kale provides iron and magnesium

"This breakfast bowl is hearty and nourishing. It keeps me full and my energy levels high."

46. Strawberry-Basil Smoothie

Ingredients:
- 1 cup fresh strawberries
- 1/2 cup coconut milk
- 1 small banana, frozen
- 1 tablespoon fresh basil leaves
- 1 teaspoon fresh lemon juice

Instructions:
1. In a blender, combine strawberries, coconut milk, banana, basil leaves, and lemon juice.
2. Blend until smooth.
3. Pour into a glass and enjoy immediately.

Health Problems Addressed: Inflammation, nutrient deficiencies

Health Benefits: Rich in vitamins and antioxidants

Scientific Benefits: Strawberries are high in vitamin C; basil has anti-inflammatory properties

"This smoothie is refreshing and unique. It's a great way to start my day with a burst of flavor and nutrients."

47. Cinnamon-Spiced Plantain Pancakes

Ingredients:
- 1 ripe plantain, peeled and mashed
- 2 eggs
- 1/4 cup coconut flour
- 1/2 teaspoon ground cinnamon
- 1/4 teaspoon baking soda
- Coconut oil for frying

Instructions:

1. In a bowl, mix mashed plantain, eggs, coconut flour, cinnamon, and baking soda.
2. In a skillet, heat coconut oil over medium heat.
3. Pour batter into the skillet to form small pancakes.
4. Cook for 2-3 minutes on each side until golden brown.
5. Serve warm.

Health Problems Addressed: Inflammation, nutrient deficiencies

Health Benefits: High in vitamins and anti-inflammatory compounds

Scientific Benefits: Plantains are rich in potassium and fiber; cinnamon has anti-inflammatory properties

"These pancakes are delicious and filling. They're a great way to enjoy a comforting breakfast while staying healthy."

48. Spinach and Mushroom Breakfast Stir-Fry

Ingredients:
- 1 tablespoon coconut oil
- 1 small onion, diced
- 1 cup mushrooms, sliced
- 2 cups spinach leaves

- 1/2 teaspoon garlic powder
- Sea salt and black pepper to taste

Instructions:
1. In a skillet, heat coconut oil over medium heat. Add onion and cook until translucent.
2. Add mushrooms and cook for 5-7 minutes until tender.
3. Add spinach leaves and cook until wilted.
4. Season with garlic powder, salt, and pepper.
5. Serve warm.

Health Problems Addressed: Inflammation, nutrient deficiencies

Health Benefits: High in vitamins, antioxidants, and anti-inflammatory compounds

Scientific Benefits: Spinach is rich in iron and magnesium; mushrooms provide B vitamins and antioxidants

"This stir-fry is flavorful and nutritious. It's a great way to start my day with a boost of vitamins and minerals."

49. Carrot and Parsnip Breakfast Bake

Ingredients:

- 1 tablespoon coconut oil
- 1 small onion, diced
- 2 carrots, peeled and grated
- 2 parsnips, peeled and grated
- 4 eggs
- Sea salt and black pepper to taste
- Fresh parsley, for garnish

Instructions:
1. Preheat the oven to 375°F (190°C).
2. In a skillet, heat coconut oil over medium heat. Add onion and cook until translucent.
3. Add grated carrots and parsnips and cook for 5 minutes until slightly tender.
4. Transfer the mixture to a greased baking dish.
5. In a bowl, whisk eggs, salt, and pepper. Pour over the vegetable mixture.
6. Bake for 25-30 minutes until eggs are fully set.
7. Garnish with fresh parsley before serving.

Health Problems Addressed: Inflammation, nutrient deficiencies

Health Benefits: High in vitamins, antioxidants, and anti-inflammatory compounds

Scientific Benefits: Carrots and parsnips are rich in vitamins A and C; eggs provide protein and essential nutrients

"This bake is hearty and delicious. It keeps me full and provides a great start to my day."

50. Pear and Ginger Breakfast Smoothie

Ingredients:
- 1 ripe pear, cored and chopped
- 1/2 cup coconut milk
- 1 small banana, frozen
- 1/2 teaspoon fresh ginger, grated
- 1 tablespoon chia seeds
- 1 teaspoon fresh lemon juice

Instructions:
1. In a blender, combine pear, coconut milk, banana, ginger, chia seeds, and lemon juice.
2. Blend until smooth.
3. Pour into a glass and enjoy immediately.

Health Problems Addressed: Inflammation, digestive health

Health Benefits: Anti-inflammatory and rich in fiber and antioxidants

Scientific Benefits: Pears are high in fiber; ginger has strong anti-inflammatory properties

"This smoothie is both soothing and energizing. It helps with my digestion and keeps me feeling refreshed."

By starting your day with these nutrient-dense, anti-inflammatory breakfasts, you can set a positive tone for the rest of your day. These recipes are designed to support your immune system, reduce inflammation, and provide sustained energy, helping you to manage your autoimmune condition effectively.

Chapter 3: Energizing Lunches

51. Grilled Chicken and Avocado Salad

Ingredients:
- 2 cups mixed greens
- 1 grilled chicken breast, sliced
- 1/2 avocado, sliced
- 1/2 cup cherry tomatoes, halved
- 1/4 cup red onion, thinly sliced
- 1 tablespoon olive oil
- 1 tablespoon fresh lemon juice
- Sea salt and black pepper to taste

Instructions:
1. In a large bowl, combine mixed greens, grilled chicken, avocado, cherry tomatoes, and red onion.
2. Drizzle with olive oil and lemon juice.
3. Season with salt and pepper, then toss to combine.
4. Serve immediately.

Health Problems Addressed: Inflammation, nutrient deficiencies

Health Benefits: High in protein, vitamins, and healthy fats

Scientific Benefits: Avocado provides healthy fats; chicken is a lean protein source

"This salad is satisfying and energizing. It keeps me full and provides the nutrients I need."

52. Sweet Potato and Kale Salad

Ingredients:
- 1 large sweet potato, peeled and cubed
- 2 tablespoons olive oil, divided
- 2 cups kale leaves, chopped
- 1/4 cup pumpkin seeds
- 1 tablespoon balsamic vinegar
- Sea salt and black pepper to taste

Instructions:
1. Preheat the oven to 400°F (200°C).
2. Toss sweet potato cubes with 1 tablespoon olive oil and spread on a baking sheet.
3. Roast for 20-25 minutes until tender and slightly browned.
4. In a large bowl, massage kale leaves with the remaining olive oil until slightly wilted.

5. Add roasted sweet potato, pumpkin seeds, and balsamic vinegar.
6. Season with salt and pepper, then toss to combine.
7. Serve immediately.

Health Problems Addressed: Inflammation, nutrient deficiencies

Health Benefits: High in vitamins and antioxidants

Scientific Benefits: Sweet potatoes are rich in vitamins A and C; kale provides iron and magnesium

"This salad is both hearty and healthy. It's a perfect midday meal that keeps me energized."

53. Zucchini Noodles with Pesto and Shrimp

Ingredients:
- 2 medium zucchinis, spiralized into noodles
- 1 tablespoon olive oil
- 1 garlic clove, minced
- 1/2 pound shrimp, peeled and deveined
- 1/4 cup basil pesto (AIP-friendly)
- Sea salt and black pepper to taste
- Fresh basil leaves, for garnish

Instructions:

1. In a large skillet, heat olive oil over medium heat. Add garlic and cook until fragrant.
2. Add shrimp and cook for 2-3 minutes on each side until pink and cooked through.
3. Add zucchini noodles and cook for 2-3 minutes until slightly tender.
4. Remove from heat and toss with basil pesto.
5. Season with salt and pepper.
6. Garnish with fresh basil leaves before serving.

Health Problems Addressed: Inflammation, nutrient deficiencies

Health Benefits: High in protein, healthy fats, and antioxidants

Scientific Benefits: Shrimp is a lean protein source; zucchini is low in calories and high in fiber

"This dish is light and flavorful. It's a great lunch that keeps me satisfied without feeling heavy."

54. Turkey and Spinach Stuffed Bell Peppers

Ingredients:
- 4 bell peppers, halved and seeds removed
- 1 tablespoon coconut oil
- 1 small onion, diced

- 1 cup cooked ground turkey
- 2 cups spinach leaves, chopped
- 1/2 teaspoon dried oregano
- Sea salt and black pepper to taste
- Fresh parsley, for garnish

Instructions:
1. Preheat the oven to 375°F (190°C).
2. In a skillet, heat coconut oil over medium heat. Add onion and cook until translucent.
3. Add cooked ground turkey and chopped spinach. Cook until spinach is wilted.
4. Season with dried oregano, salt, and pepper.
5. Stuffed bell pepper halves with the turkey and spinach mixture.
6. Place stuffed peppers in a baking dish and bake for 25-30 minutes until peppers are tender.
7. Garnish with fresh parsley before serving.

Health Problems Addressed: Inflammation, nutrient deficiencies

Health Benefits: High in protein and vitamins

Scientific Benefits: Bell peppers are rich in vitamins A and C; spinach provides iron and magnesium

"These stuffed peppers are delicious and filling. They make a great lunch that keeps me going all afternoon."

55. Salmon and Avocado Lettuce Wraps

Ingredients:
- 4 large lettuce leaves
- 1 cooked salmon fillet, flaked
- 1/2 avocado, sliced
- 1/4 cup cucumber, sliced
- 1 tablespoon fresh lemon juice
- Sea salt and black pepper to taste

Instructions:
1. Lay out lettuce leaves on a flat surface.
2. Divide flaked salmon, avocado slices, and cucumber slices evenly among the lettuce leaves.
3. Drizzle with fresh lemon juice.
4. Season with salt and pepper.
5. Roll up the lettuce leaves to form wraps.
6. Serve immediately.

Health Problems Addressed: Inflammation, nutrient deficiencies

Health Benefits: High in omega-3 fatty acids and healthy fats

Scientific Benefits: Salmon provides omega-3 fatty acids; avocado is rich in healthy fats

"These lettuce wraps are fresh and light. They're perfect for a quick and healthy lunch."

56. Cucumber and Dill Chicken Salad

Ingredients:
- 2 cups cooked chicken breast, shredded
- 1/2 cucumber, diced
- 1/4 cup red onion, diced
- 1/4 cup coconut yogurt
- 1 tablespoon fresh dill, chopped
- 1 tablespoon fresh lemon juice
- Sea salt and black pepper to taste

Instructions:
1. In a large bowl, combine shredded chicken, diced cucumber, and red onion.
2. In a small bowl, mix coconut yogurt, fresh dill, lemon juice, salt, and pepper.
3. Pour the dressing over the chicken mixture and toss to combine.
4. Serve immediately or refrigerate until ready to eat.

Health Problems Addressed: Inflammation, nutrient deficiencies

Health Benefits: High in protein and vitamins

Scientific Benefits: Chicken is a lean protein source; cucumber is hydrating and rich in antioxidants

"This chicken salad is refreshing and flavorful. It's a great way to enjoy a healthy lunch."

57. Beet and Carrot Slaw

Ingredients:
- 1 large beet, peeled and grated
- 2 large carrots, peeled and grated
- 1/4 cup fresh cilantro, chopped
- 2 tablespoons olive oil
- 1 tablespoon apple cider vinegar
- Sea salt and black pepper to taste

Instructions:
1. In a large bowl, combine grated beet, grated carrots, and fresh cilantro.
2. In a small bowl, whisk together olive oil, apple cider vinegar, salt, and pepper.
3. Pour the dressing over the slaw and toss to combine.
4. Serve immediately or refrigerate until ready to eat.

Health Problems Addressed: Inflammation, nutrient deficiencies

Health Benefits: High in antioxidants and fiber

Scientific Benefits: Beets and carrots are rich in vitamins A and C; apple cider vinegar aids digestion

"This slaw is crunchy and vibrant. It's a perfect side dish for any meal."

58. Cauliflower and Broccoli Rice Bowl

Ingredients:
- 1 tablespoon coconut oil
- 1 small onion, diced
- 1 cup cauliflower rice
- 1 cup broccoli rice
- 1/2 teaspoon turmeric
- Sea salt and black pepper to taste
- Fresh parsley, for garnish

Instructions:
1. In a skillet, heat coconut oil over medium heat. Add onion and cook until translucent.
2. Add cauliflower rice and broccoli rice, and cook for 5-7 minutes until tender.
3. Season with turmeric, salt, and pepper.

4. Garnish with fresh parsley before serving.

Health Problems Addressed: Inflammation, nutrient deficiencies

Health Benefits: High in fiber, vitamins, and anti-inflammatory compounds

Scientific Benefits: Cauliflower and broccoli are rich in vitamins C and K; turmeric has anti-inflammatory properties

"This rice bowl is hearty and nutritious. It's a great way to enjoy a filling lunch without grains."

59. Avocado and Bacon Salad

Ingredients:
- 2 cups mixed greens
- 1/2 avocado, sliced
- 4 slices cooked bacon, crumbled
- 1/4 cup red onion, thinly sliced
- 1 tablespoon olive oil
- 1 tablespoon fresh lemon juice
- Sea salt and black pepper to taste

Instructions:

1. In a large bowl, combine mixed greens, avocado slices, crumbled bacon, and red onion.
2. Drizzle with olive oil and lemon juice.
3. Season with salt and pepper, then toss to combine.
4. Serve immediately.

Health Problems Addressed: Inflammation, nutrient deficiencies

Health Benefits: High in healthy fats and protein

Scientific Benefits: Avocado provides healthy fats; bacon in moderation adds flavor and protein

"This salad is savory and satisfying. It's a perfect balance of flavors and textures."

60. Ginger-Turmeric Chicken Soup

Ingredients:
- 1 tablespoon coconut oil
- 1 small onion, diced
- 2 garlic cloves, minced
- 1 inch fresh ginger, grated
- 1 teaspoon ground turmeric
- 4 cups chicken broth
- 1 cup cooked shredded chicken
- 1 cup carrots, sliced

- 1 cup spinach leaves
- Sea salt and black pepper to taste

Instructions:
1. In a large pot, heat coconut oil over medium heat. Add onion and cook until translucent.
2. Add garlic, ginger, and turmeric, and cook for 1-2 minutes until fragrant.
3. Add chicken broth, shredded chicken, and carrots. Bring to a simmer.
4. Cook for 10-15 minutes until carrots are tender.
5. Add spinach leaves and cook until wilted.
6. Season with salt and pepper before serving.

Health Problems Addressed: Inflammation, digestive health

Health Benefits: Anti-inflammatory and rich in protein and vitamins

Scientific Benefits: Turmeric and ginger have strong anti-inflammatory properties; chicken provides lean protein

"This soup is comforting and healing. It's my go-to lunch when I need a boost."

61. Basil and Tomato Tuna Salad

Ingredients:
- 2 cans tuna in water, drained
- 1/2 cup cherry tomatoes, halved
- 1/4 cup fresh basil leaves, chopped
- 2 tablespoons olive oil
- 1 tablespoon fresh lemon juice
- Sea salt and black pepper to taste

Instructions:
1. In a large bowl, combine drained tuna, cherry tomatoes, and fresh basil.
2. Drizzle with olive oil and lemon juice.
3. Season with salt and pepper, then toss to combine.
4. Serve immediately or refrigerate until ready to eat.

Health Problems Addressed: Inflammation, nutrient deficiencies

Health Benefits: High in protein and omega-3 fatty acids

Scientific Benefits: Tuna provides lean protein and omega-3s; tomatoes are rich in antioxidants

"This tuna salad is fresh and delicious. It's a perfect lunch that's easy to make and nutritious."

62. Coconut Curry Chicken

Ingredients:
- 1 tablespoon coconut oil
- 1 small onion, diced
- 2 garlic cloves, minced
- 1 tablespoon curry powder
- 1 can coconut milk
- 2 cups cooked chicken breast, shredded
- 1 cup carrots, sliced
- Sea salt and black pepper to taste
- Fresh cilantro, for garnish

Instructions:
1. In a large pot, heat coconut oil over medium heat. Add onion and cook until translucent.
2. Add garlic and curry powder, and cook for 1-2 minutes until fragrant.
3. Add coconut milk, shredded chicken, and carrots. Bring to a simmer.
4. Cook for 10-15 minutes until carrots are tender.
5. Season with salt and pepper.
6. Garnish with fresh cilantro before serving.

Health Problems Addressed: Inflammation, nutrient deficiencies

Health Benefits: Anti-inflammatory and rich in protein and vitamins

Scientific Benefits: Curry powder has anti-inflammatory properties; coconut milk provides healthy fats

"This curry is flavorful and satisfying. It's a comforting lunch that keeps me full and happy."

63. Roasted Vegetable and Chicken Bowl

Ingredients:
- 1 tablespoon olive oil
- 1 small sweet potato, peeled and cubed
- 1 cup broccoli florets
- 1 cup cauliflower florets
- 1 cup cooked chicken breast, sliced
- 1 tablespoon balsamic vinegar
- Sea salt and black pepper to taste

Instructions:
1. Preheat the oven to 400°F (200°C).
2. Toss sweet potato cubes, broccoli florets, and cauliflower florets with olive oil. Spread on a baking sheet.
3. Roast for 20-25 minutes until tender and slightly browned.
4. In a bowl, combine roasted vegetables and sliced chicken.

5. Drizzle with balsamic vinegar and season with salt and pepper.

6. Toss to combine and serve immediately.

Health Problems Addressed: Inflammation, nutrient deficiencies

Health Benefits: High in vitamins, antioxidants, and protein

Scientific Benefits: Sweet potatoes and broccoli are rich in vitamins A and C; chicken provides lean protein

"This bowl is hearty and nutritious. It's a perfect lunch that's easy to prepare and delicious."

64. Spinach and Apple Salad with Poppy Seed Dressing

Ingredients:
- 2 cups spinach leaves
- 1 apple, sliced
- 1/4 cup red onion, thinly sliced
- 1/4 cup walnuts, chopped
- 2 tablespoons olive oil
- 1 tablespoon apple cider vinegar
- 1 teaspoon poppy seeds
- Sea salt and black pepper to taste

Instructions:
1. In a large bowl, combine spinach leaves, apple slices, red onion, and chopped walnuts.
2. In a small bowl, whisk together olive oil, apple cider vinegar, poppy seeds, salt, and pepper.
3. Drizzle the dressing over the salad and toss to combine.
4. Serve immediately.

Health Problems Addressed: Inflammation, nutrient deficiencies

Health Benefits: High in vitamins, healthy fats, and antioxidants

Scientific Benefits: Spinach is rich in iron and magnesium; apples are high in fiber and antioxidants

"This salad is fresh and crunchy. It's a delicious and healthy lunch option."

65. Cucumber and Dill Salmon Salad

Ingredients:
- 2 cups mixed greens
- 1 cooked salmon fillet, flaked
- 1/2 cucumber, diced

- 1/4 cup red onion, diced
- 1/4 cup coconut yogurt
- 1 tablespoon fresh dill, chopped
- 1 tablespoon fresh lemon juice
- Sea salt and black pepper to taste

Instructions:

1. In a large bowl, combine mixed greens, flaked salmon, diced cucumber, and red onion.
2. In a small bowl, mix coconut yogurt, fresh dill, lemon juice, salt, and pepper.
3. Pour the dressing over the salad and toss to combine.
4. Serve immediately or refrigerate until ready to eat.

Health Problems Addressed: Inflammation, nutrient deficiencies

Health Benefits: High in omega-3 fatty acids, protein, and vitamins

Scientific Benefits: Salmon provides omega-3 fatty acids; cucumber is hydrating and rich in antioxidants

"This salmon salad is refreshing and satisfying. It's a perfect lunch that's both healthy and tasty."

66. Roasted Butternut Squash and Brussels Sprouts Salad

Ingredients:
- 1 small butternut squash, peeled and cubed
- 1 cup Brussels sprouts, halved
- 2 tablespoons olive oil
- 2 cups mixed greens
- 1/4 cup pomegranate seeds
- 1 tablespoon balsamic vinegar
- Sea salt and black pepper to taste

Instructions:
1. Preheat the oven to 400°F (200°C).
2. Toss butternut squash cubes and Brussels sprouts with olive oil. Spread on a baking sheet.
3. Roast for 20-25 minutes until tender and slightly browned.
4. In a large bowl, combine mixed greens, roasted butternut squash, and Brussels sprouts.
5. Add pomegranate seeds and drizzle with balsamic vinegar.
6. Season with salt and pepper, then toss to combine.
7. Serve immediately.

Health Problems Addressed: Inflammation, nutrient deficiencies

Health Benefits: High in vitamins, antioxidants, and fiber

Scientific Benefits: Butternut squash and Brussels sprouts are rich in vitamins A and C; pomegranate seeds are high in antioxidants

"This salad is colorful and delicious. It's a great way to enjoy a healthy and satisfying lunch."

67. Turkey and Avocado Lettuce Wraps

Ingredients:
- 4 large lettuce leaves
- 1 cup cooked ground turkey
- 1/2 avocado, sliced
- 1/4 cup red onion, diced
- 1 tablespoon fresh lime juice
- Sea salt and black pepper to taste

Instructions:
1. Lay out lettuce leaves on a flat surface.
2. Divide cooked ground turkey, avocado slices, and red onion evenly among the lettuce leaves.
3. Drizzle with fresh lime juice.
4. Season with salt and pepper.
5. Roll up the lettuce leaves to form wraps.
6. Serve immediately.

Health Problems Addressed: Inflammation, nutrient deficiencies

Health Benefits: High in protein and healthy fats

Scientific Benefits: Turkey provides lean protein; avocado is rich in healthy fats

"These lettuce wraps are light and delicious. They're perfect for a quick and healthy lunch."

68. Cauliflower and Sweet Potato Soup

Ingredients:
- 1 tablespoon coconut oil
- 1 small onion, diced
- 2 garlic cloves, minced
- 1 large sweet potato, peeled and cubed
- 1 head cauliflower, chopped
- 4 cups vegetable broth
- 1/2 teaspoon ground cumin
- Sea salt and black pepper to taste
- Fresh cilantro, for garnish

Instructions:
1. In a large pot, heat coconut oil over medium heat. Add onion and cook until translucent.

2. Add garlic, sweet potato, and cauliflower, and cook for 5-7 minutes.

3. Add vegetable broth and bring to a simmer.

4. Cook for 20-25 minutes until vegetables are tender.

5. Use an immersion blender to puree the soup until smooth.

6. Season with ground cumin, salt, and pepper.

7. Garnish with fresh cilantro before serving.

Health Problems Addressed: Inflammation, nutrient deficiencies

Health Benefits: High in vitamins, fiber, and antioxidants

Scientific Benefits: Sweet potatoes and cauliflower are rich in vitamins A and C; cumin has anti-inflammatory properties

"This soup is creamy and comforting. It's a perfect lunch that's both filling and nutritious."

69. Chicken and Zucchini Stir-Fry

Ingredients:
- 1 tablespoon coconut oil
- 1 small onion, diced
- 2 garlic cloves, minced
- 1 cup cooked chicken breast, sliced

- 2 medium zucchinis, sliced
- 1 red bell pepper, sliced
- 1 tablespoon coconut aminos
- Sea salt and black pepper to taste
- Fresh basil leaves, for garnish

Instructions:
1. In a large skillet, heat coconut oil over medium heat. Add onion and cook until translucent.
2. Add garlic and cook for 1-2 minutes until fragrant.
3. Add sliced chicken, zucchinis, and bell pepper. Cook for 5-7 minutes until vegetables are tender.
4. Drizzle with coconut aminos and season with salt and pepper.
5. Garnish with fresh basil leaves before serving.

Health Problems Addressed: Inflammation, nutrient deficiencies

Health Benefits: High in protein and vitamins

Scientific Benefits: Zucchini is low in calories and high in fiber; chicken provides lean protein

"This stir-fry is quick and easy. It's a great lunch that's both healthy and delicious."

70. Beet and Arugula Salad with Citrus Dressing

Ingredients:
- 2 cups arugula leaves
- 1 large beet, peeled and grated
- 1/2 orange, peeled and segmented
- 1/4 cup walnuts, chopped
- 2 tablespoons olive oil
- 1 tablespoon fresh orange juice
- Sea salt and black pepper to taste

Instructions:
1. In a large bowl, combine arugula leaves, grated beet, orange segments, and chopped walnuts.
2. In a small bowl, whisk together olive oil, fresh orange juice, salt, and pepper.
3. Drizzle the dressing over the salad and toss to combine.
4. Serve immediately.

Health Problems Addressed: Inflammation, nutrient deficiencies

Health Benefits: High in vitamins, antioxidants, and healthy fats

Scientific Benefits: Beets and oranges are rich in vitamins A and C; arugula provides iron and magnesium

"This salad is bright and refreshing. It's a delicious and healthy lunch option."

71. Turkey and Cranberry Salad

Ingredients:
- 2 cups mixed greens
- 1 cup cooked turkey breast, sliced
- 1/4 cup dried cranberries (unsweetened)
- 1/4 cup walnuts, chopped
- 2 tablespoons olive oil
- 1 tablespoon balsamic vinegar
- Sea salt and black pepper to taste

Instructions:
1. In a large bowl, combine mixed greens, sliced turkey, dried cranberries, and walnuts.
2. Drizzle with olive oil and balsamic vinegar.
3. Season with salt and pepper, then toss to combine.
4. Serve immediately.

Health Problems Addressed: Inflammation, nutrient deficiencies

Health Benefits: High in protein, healthy fats, and antioxidants

Scientific Benefits: Turkey provides lean protein; cranberries are rich in antioxidants

"This salad is festive and satisfying. It's a great way to enjoy leftover turkey."

72. Shrimp and Mango Salad

Ingredients:
- 2 cups mixed greens
- 1/2 cup cooked shrimp, peeled and deveined
- 1/2 mango, diced
- 1/4 cup red bell pepper, diced
- 2 tablespoons olive oil
- 1 tablespoon fresh lime juice
- Sea salt and black pepper to taste

Instructions:
1. In a large bowl, combine mixed greens, cooked shrimp, mango, and red bell pepper.
2. Drizzle with olive oil and fresh lime juice.
3. Season with salt and pepper, then toss to combine.
4. Serve immediately.

Health Problems Addressed: Inflammation, nutrient deficiencies

Health Benefits: High in protein, vitamins, and antioxidants

Scientific Benefits: Shrimp is a lean protein source; mango is rich in vitamins A and C

"This salad is light and refreshing. The mango adds a sweet and tropical flavor."

73. Beef and Broccoli Stir-Fry

Ingredients:
- 1 tablespoon coconut oil
- 1 small onion, diced
- 1 garlic clove, minced
- 1 cup cooked beef, sliced
- 2 cups broccoli florets
- 1 tablespoon coconut aminos
- Sea salt and black pepper to taste
- Fresh cilantro, for garnish

Instructions:
1. In a large skillet, heat coconut oil over medium heat. Add onion and cook until translucent.
2. Add garlic and cook for 1-2 minutes until fragrant.
3. Add sliced beef and broccoli florets. Cook for 5-7 minutes until broccoli is tender.

4. Drizzle with coconut aminos and season with salt and pepper.
5. Garnish with fresh cilantro before serving.

Health Problems Addressed: Inflammation, nutrient deficiencies

Health Benefits: High in protein and vitamins

Scientific Benefits: Broccoli is rich in vitamins C and K; beef provides iron and protein

"This stir-fry is savory and satisfying. It's a quick and nutritious lunch."

74. Tuna and Avocado Salad

Ingredients:
- 2 cans tuna in water, drained
- 1/2 avocado, diced
- 1/4 cup red onion, diced
- 1 tablespoon fresh lemon juice
- Sea salt and black pepper to taste

Instructions:
1. In a large bowl, combine drained tuna, diced avocado, and red onion.
2. Drizzle with fresh lemon juice.

3. Season with salt and pepper, then toss to combine.
4. Serve immediately.

Health Problems Addressed: Inflammation, nutrient deficiencies

Health Benefits: High in protein, omega-3 fatty acids, and healthy fats

Scientific Benefits: Tuna provides lean protein and omega-3s; avocado is rich in healthy fats

"This salad is creamy and delicious. It's a perfect lunch that's both healthy and satisfying."

75. Chicken and Apple Salad

Ingredients:
- 2 cups mixed greens
- 1 cup cooked chicken breast, sliced
- 1 apple, diced
- 1/4 cup walnuts, chopped
- 2 tablespoons olive oil
- 1 tablespoon apple cider vinegar
- Sea salt and black pepper to taste

Instructions:

1. In a large bowl, combine mixed greens, sliced chicken, diced apple, and chopped walnuts.
2. Drizzle with olive oil and apple cider vinegar.
3. Season with salt and pepper, then toss to combine.
4. Serve immediately.

Health Problems Addressed: Inflammation, nutrient deficiencies

Health Benefits: High in protein, vitamins, and healthy fats

Scientific Benefits: Chicken provides lean protein; apples are rich in fiber and antioxidants

"This salad is fresh and crunchy. It's a delicious and healthy lunch option."

76. Zucchini and Tomato Salad

Ingredients:
- 2 medium zucchinis, spiralized into noodles
- 1 cup cherry tomatoes, halved
- 1/4 cup red onion, thinly sliced
- 2 tablespoons olive oil
- 1 tablespoon balsamic vinegar
- Sea salt and black pepper to taste

Instructions:

1. In a large bowl, combine zucchini noodles, cherry tomatoes, and red onion.
2. Drizzle with olive oil and balsamic vinegar.
3. Season with salt and pepper, then toss to combine.
4. Serve immediately.

Health Problems Addressed: Inflammation, nutrient deficiencies

Health Benefits: High in vitamins and antioxidants

Scientific Benefits: Zucchini is low in calories and high in fiber; tomatoes are rich in antioxidants

"This salad is light and refreshing. It's a great way to enjoy a raw and crunchy lunch."

77. Lemon Herb Chicken Salad

Ingredients:
- 2 cups mixed greens
- 1 cup cooked chicken breast, sliced
- 1/4 cup fresh herbs (parsley, cilantro, dill), chopped
- 1/4 cup cucumber, diced
- 2 tablespoons olive oil
- 1 tablespoon fresh lemon juice
- Sea salt and black pepper to taste

Instructions:
1. In a large bowl, combine mixed greens, sliced chicken, fresh herbs, and cucumber.
2. Drizzle with olive oil and fresh lemon juice.
3. Season with salt and pepper, then toss to combine.
4. Serve immediately.

Health Problems Addressed: Inflammation, nutrient deficiencies

Health Benefits: High in protein, vitamins, and antioxidants

Scientific Benefits: Herbs provide antioxidants and anti-inflammatory properties; chicken is a lean protein source

"This salad is fresh and zesty. The herbs add a burst of flavor that's delicious."

78. Beef and Avocado Lettuce Wraps

Ingredients:
- 4 large lettuce leaves
- 1 cup cooked ground beef
- 1/2 avocado, sliced
- 1/4 cup red onion, diced

- 1 tablespoon fresh lime juice
- Sea salt and black pepper to taste

Instructions:
1. Lay out lettuce leaves on a flat surface.
2. Divide cooked ground beef, avocado slices, and red onion evenly among the lettuce leaves.
3. Drizzle with fresh lime juice.
4. Season with salt and pepper.
5. Roll up the lettuce leaves to form wraps.
6. Serve immediately.

Health Problems Addressed: Inflammation, nutrient deficiencies

Health Benefits: High in protein and healthy fats

Scientific Benefits: Beef provides iron and protein; avocado is rich in healthy fats

"These lettuce wraps are hearty and delicious. They're perfect for a quick and healthy lunch."

79. Sweet Potato and Apple Salad

Ingredients:
- 1 large sweet potato, peeled and cubed
- 1 apple, diced

- 1/4 cup pecans, chopped
- 2 tablespoons olive oil
- 1 tablespoon apple cider vinegar
- Sea salt and black pepper to taste

Instructions:
1. Preheat the oven to 400°F (200°C).
2. Toss sweet potato cubes with 1 tablespoon olive oil and spread on a baking sheet.
3. Roast for 20-25 minutes until tender and slightly browned.
4. In a large bowl, combine roasted sweet potato, diced apple, and chopped pecans.
5. Drizzle with remaining olive oil and apple cider vinegar.
6. Season with salt and pepper, then toss to combine.
7. Serve immediately.

Health Problems Addressed: Inflammation, nutrient deficiencies

Health Benefits: High in vitamins, antioxidants, and healthy fats

Scientific Benefits: Sweet potatoes are rich in vitamins A and C; apples are high in fiber

"This salad is warm and comforting. The combination of sweet potato and apple is delicious."

80. Salmon and Spinach Salad

Ingredients:
- 2 cups spinach leaves
- 1 cooked salmon fillet, flaked
- 1/4 cup red onion, diced
- 1/4 cup pumpkin seeds
- 2 tablespoons olive oil
- 1 tablespoon fresh lemon juice
- Sea salt and black pepper to taste

Instructions:
1. In a large bowl, combine spinach leaves, flaked salmon, red onion, and pumpkin seeds.
2. Drizzle with olive oil and fresh lemon juice.
3. Season with salt and pepper, then toss to combine.
4. Serve immediately.

Health Problems Addressed: Inflammation, nutrient deficiencies

Health Benefits: High in omega-3 fatty acids, protein, and vitamins

Scientific Benefits: Salmon provides omega-3 fatty acids; spinach is rich in iron and magnesium

"This salad is rich and flavorful. The salmon adds a satisfying protein boost."

81. Cauliflower and Pomegranate Salad

Ingredients:
- 1 head cauliflower, chopped into florets
- 1/2 cup pomegranate seeds
- 1/4 cup red onion, diced
- 2 tablespoons olive oil
- 1 tablespoon balsamic vinegar
- Sea salt and black pepper to taste

Instructions:
1. Preheat the oven to 400°F (200°C).
2. Toss cauliflower florets with 1 tablespoon olive oil and spread on a baking sheet.
3. Roast for 20-25 minutes until tender and slightly browned.
4. In a large bowl, combine roasted cauliflower, pomegranate seeds, and red onion.
5. Drizzle with remaining olive oil and balsamic vinegar.
6. Season with salt and pepper, then toss to combine.
7. Serve immediately.

Health Problems Addressed: Inflammation, nutrient deficiencies

Health Benefits: High in vitamins, antioxidants, and fiber

Scientific Benefits: Cauliflower is rich in vitamins C and K; pomegranate seeds are high in antioxidants

"This salad is vibrant and delicious. The pomegranate seeds add a sweet and tangy touch."

82. Turkey and Sweet Potato Hash

Ingredients:
- 1 tablespoon coconut oil
- 1 small onion, diced
- 2 garlic cloves, minced
- 1 large sweet potato, peeled and diced
- 1 cup cooked turkey breast, diced
- Sea salt and black pepper to taste
- Fresh parsley, for garnish

Instructions:
1. In a large skillet, heat coconut oil over medium heat. Add onion and cook until translucent.
2. Add garlic and cook for 1-2 minutes until fragrant.

3. Add diced sweet potato and cook for 10-15 minutes until tender.

4. Add cooked turkey and cook until heated through.

5. Season with salt and pepper.

6. Garnish with fresh parsley before serving.

Health Problems Addressed: Inflammation, nutrient deficiencies

Health Benefits: High in protein, vitamins, and antioxidants

Scientific Benefits: Sweet potatoes are rich in vitamins A and C; turkey provides lean protein

"This hash is hearty and filling. It's a perfect lunch that's both nutritious and tasty."

83. Shrimp and Avocado Salad

Ingredients:
- 2 cups mixed greens
- 1/2 cup cooked shrimp, peeled and deveined
- 1/2 avocado, sliced
- 1/4 cup cherry tomatoes, halved
- 2 tablespoons olive oil
- 1 tablespoon fresh lime juice
- Sea salt and black pepper to taste

Instructions:
1. In a large bowl, combine mixed greens, cooked shrimp, avocado slices, and cherry tomatoes.
2. Drizzle with olive oil and fresh lime juice.
3. Season with salt and pepper, then toss to combine.
4. Serve immediately.

Health Problems Addressed: Inflammation, nutrient deficiencies

Health Benefits: High in protein, healthy fats, and vitamins

Scientific Benefits: Shrimp is a lean protein source; avocado is rich in healthy fats

"This salad is light and refreshing. It's a great lunch option that's both healthy and delicious."

84. Chicken and Kale Soup

Ingredients:
- 1 tablespoon coconut oil
- 1 small onion, diced
- 2 garlic cloves, minced
- 1 cup cooked chicken breast, shredded
- 4 cups chicken broth

- 2 cups kale leaves, chopped
- Sea salt and black pepper to taste

Instructions:
1. In a large pot, heat coconut oil over medium heat. Add onion and cook until translucent.
2. Add garlic and cook for 1-2 minutes until fragrant.
3. Add shredded chicken and chicken broth. Bring to a simmer.
4. Add chopped kale and cook until wilted.
5. Season with salt and pepper before serving.

Health Problems Addressed: Inflammation, nutrient deficiencies

Health Benefits: High in protein, vitamins, and antioxidants

Scientific Benefits: Kale is rich in vitamins A and C; chicken provides lean protein

"This soup is hearty and nourishing. It's a perfect lunch to keep me warm and satisfied."

85. Salmon and Cucumber Salad

Ingredients:
- 2 cups mixed greens

- 1 cooked salmon fillet, flaked
- 1/2 cucumber, diced
- 1/4 cup red onion, diced
- 2 tablespoons olive oil
- 1 tablespoon fresh lemon juice
- Sea salt and black pepper to taste

Instructions:
1. In a large bowl, combine mixed greens, flaked salmon, diced cucumber, and red onion.
2. Drizzle with olive oil and fresh lemon juice.
3. Season with salt and pepper, then toss to combine.
4. Serve immediately.

Health Problems Addressed: Inflammation, nutrient deficiencies

Health Benefits: High in omega-3 fatty acids, protein, and vitamins

Scientific Benefits: Salmon provides omega-3 fatty acids; cucumber is hydrating and rich in antioxidants

"This salad is refreshing and satisfying. It's a perfect lunch that's both healthy and tasty."

86. Beef and Sweet Potato Salad

Ingredients:
- 1 large sweet potato, peeled and cubed
- 1 cup cooked beef, sliced
- 2 cups mixed greens
- 1/4 cup cherry tomatoes, halved
- 2 tablespoons olive oil
- 1 tablespoon balsamic vinegar
- Sea salt and black pepper to taste

Instructions:
1. Preheat the oven to 400°F (200°C).
2. Toss sweet potato cubes with 1 tablespoon olive oil and spread on a baking sheet.
3. Roast for 20-25 minutes until tender and slightly browned.
4. In a large bowl, combine roasted sweet potato, sliced beef, mixed greens, and cherry tomatoes.
5. Drizzle with remaining olive oil and balsamic vinegar.
6. Season with salt and pepper, then toss to combine.
7. Serve immediately.

Health Problems Addressed: Inflammation, nutrient deficiencies

Health Benefits: High in protein, vitamins, and antioxidants

Scientific Benefits: Sweet potatoes are rich in vitamins A and C; beef provides iron and protein

"This salad is hearty and flavorful. It's a great lunch that's both filling and nutritious."

87. Chicken and Mango Salad

Ingredients:
- 2 cups mixed greens
- 1 cup cooked chicken breast, sliced
- 1/2 mango, diced
- 1/4 cup red onion, diced
- 2 tablespoons olive oil
- 1 tablespoon fresh lime juice
- Sea salt and black pepper to taste

Instructions:
1. In a large bowl, combine mixed greens, sliced chicken, diced mango, and red onion.
2. Drizzle with olive oil and fresh lime juice.
3. Season with salt and pepper, then toss to combine.
4. Serve immediately.

Health Problems Addressed: Inflammation, nutrient deficiencies

Health Benefits: High in protein, vitamins, and antioxidants

Scientific Benefits: Mango is rich in vitamins A and C; chicken provides lean protein

"This salad is tropical and delicious. The mango adds a sweet and juicy flavor."

88. Cauliflower and Chicken Soup

Ingredients:
- 1 tablespoon coconut oil
- 1 small onion, diced
- 2 garlic cloves, minced
- 1 head cauliflower, chopped
- 1 cup cooked chicken breast, shredded
- 4 cups chicken broth
- Sea salt and black pepper to taste

Instructions:
1. In a large pot, heat coconut oil over medium heat. Add onion and cook until translucent.
2. Add garlic and cook for 1-2 minutes until fragrant.
3. Add chopped cauliflower and cook for 5-7 minutes.
4. Add chicken broth and bring to a simmer.
5. Cook for 20-25 minutes until cauliflower is tender.

6. Use an immersion blender to puree the soup until smooth.

7. Add shredded chicken and cook until heated through.

8. Season with salt and pepper before serving.

Health Problems Addressed: Inflammation, nutrient deficiencies

Health Benefits: High in vitamins, fiber, and protein

Scientific Benefits: Cauliflower is rich in vitamins C and K; chicken provides lean protein

"This soup is creamy and comforting. It's a perfect lunch that's both filling and nutritious."

89. Shrimp and Pineapple Salad

Ingredients:
- 2 cups mixed greens
- 1/2 cup cooked shrimp, peeled and deveined
- 1/2 cup pineapple chunks
- 1/4 cup red bell pepper, diced
- 2 tablespoons olive oil
- 1 tablespoon fresh lime juice
- Sea salt and black pepper to taste

Instructions:

1. In a large bowl, combine mixed greens, cooked shrimp, pineapple chunks, and red bell pepper.
2. Drizzle with olive oil and fresh lime juice.
3. Season with salt and pepper, then toss to combine.
4. Serve immediately.

Health Problems Addressed: Inflammation, nutrient deficiencies

Health Benefits: High in protein, vitamins, and antioxidants

Scientific Benefits: Pineapple is rich in vitamin C; shrimp provides lean protein

"This salad is sweet and refreshing. It's a great lunch option that's both healthy and delicious."

90. Turkey and Cranberry Lettuce Wraps

Ingredients:
- 4 large lettuce leaves
- 1 cup cooked turkey breast, sliced
- 1/4 cup dried cranberries (unsweetened)
- 1/4 cup walnuts, chopped
- 2 tablespoons olive oil
- Sea salt and black pepper to taste

Instructions:
1. Lay out lettuce leaves on a flat surface.
2. Divide sliced turkey, dried cranberries, and walnuts evenly among the lettuce leaves.
3. Drizzle with olive oil.
4. Season with salt and pepper.
5. Roll up the lettuce leaves to form wraps.
6. Serve immediately.

Health Problems Addressed: Inflammation, nutrient deficiencies

Health Benefits: High in protein, healthy fats, and antioxidants

Scientific Benefits: Turkey provides lean protein; cranberries are rich in antioxidants

"These lettuce wraps are festive and satisfying. They're a great way to enjoy leftover turkey."

91. Chicken and Avocado Lettuce Wraps

Ingredients:
- 4 large lettuce leaves
- 1 cup cooked chicken breast, sliced
- 1/2 avocado, sliced
- 1/4 cup red onion, diced

- 1 tablespoon fresh lime juice
- Sea salt and black pepper to taste

Instructions:
1. Lay out lettuce leaves on a flat surface.
2. Divide sliced chicken, avocado, and red onion evenly among the lettuce leaves.
3. Drizzle with fresh lime juice.
4. Season with salt and pepper.
5. Roll up the lettuce leaves to form wraps.
6. Serve immediately.

Health Problems Addressed: Inflammation, nutrient deficiencies

Health Benefits: High in protein and healthy fats

Scientific Benefits: Chicken provides lean protein; avocado is rich in healthy fats

"These lettuce wraps are creamy and delicious. They're a perfect lunch option that's both healthy and satisfying."

92. Beef and Apple Salad

Ingredients:
- 2 cups mixed greens
- 1 cup cooked beef, sliced

- 1 apple, diced
- 1/4 cup walnuts, chopped
- 2 tablespoons olive oil
- 1 tablespoon apple cider vinegar
- Sea salt and black pepper to taste

Instructions:

1. In a large bowl, combine mixed greens, sliced beef, diced apple, and chopped walnuts.
2. Drizzle with olive oil and apple cider vinegar.
3. Season with salt and pepper, then toss to combine.
4. Serve immediately.

Health Problems Addressed: Inflammation, nutrient deficiencies

Health Benefits: High in protein, vitamins, and healthy fats

Scientific Benefits: Beef provides iron and protein; apples are rich in fiber and antioxidants

"This salad is fresh and crunchy. It's a delicious and healthy lunch option."

93. Tuna and Avocado Lettuce Wraps

Ingredients:

- 4 large lettuce leaves
- 2 cans tuna in water, drained
- 1/2 avocado, sliced
- 1/4 cup red onion, diced
- 1 tablespoon fresh lemon juice
- Sea salt and black pepper to taste

Instructions:
1. Lay out lettuce leaves on a flat surface.
2. Divide drained tuna, avocado slices, and red onion evenly among the lettuce leaves.
3. Drizzle with fresh lemon juice.
4. Season with salt and pepper.
5. Roll up the lettuce leaves to form wraps.
6. Serve immediately.

Health Problems Addressed: Inflammation, nutrient deficiencies

Health Benefits: High in protein, omega-3 fatty acids, and healthy fats

Scientific Benefits: Tuna provides lean protein and omega-3s; avocado is rich in healthy fats

"These lettuce wraps are light and satisfying. They're a perfect lunch option that's both healthy and delicious."

94. Shrimp and Avocado Lettuce Wraps

Ingredients:
- 4 large lettuce leaves
- 1/2 cup cooked shrimp, peeled and deveined
- 1/2 avocado, sliced
- 1/4 cup cherry tomatoes, halved
- 1 tablespoon fresh lime juice
- Sea salt and black pepper to taste

Instructions:
1. Lay out lettuce leaves on a flat surface.
2. Divide cooked shrimp, avocado slices, and cherry tomatoes evenly among the lettuce leaves.
3. Drizzle with fresh lime juice.
4. Season with salt and pepper.
5. Roll up the lettuce leaves to form wraps.
6. Serve immediately.

Health Problems Addressed: Inflammation, nutrient deficiencies

Health Benefits: High in protein, healthy fats, and vitamins

Scientific Benefits: Shrimp is a lean protein source; avocado is rich in healthy fats

"These lettuce wraps are light and refreshing. They're a perfect lunch option that's both healthy and delicious."

95. Chicken and Pomegranate Salad

Ingredients:
- 2 cups mixed greens
- 1 cup cooked chicken breast, sliced
- 1/2 cup pomegranate seeds
- 1/4 cup red onion, diced
- 2 tablespoons olive oil
- 1 tablespoon balsamic vinegar
- Sea salt and black pepper to taste

Instructions:
1. In a large bowl, combine mixed greens, sliced chicken, pomegranate seeds, and red onion.
2. Drizzle with olive oil and balsamic vinegar.
3. Season with salt and pepper, then toss to combine.
4. Serve immediately.

Health Problems Addressed: Inflammation, nutrient deficiencies

Health Benefits: High in protein, vitamins, and antioxidants

Scientific Benefits: Pomegranate seeds are high in antioxidants; chicken provides lean protein

"This salad is vibrant and delicious. The pomegranate seeds add a sweet and tangy touch."

96. Turkey and Avocado Salad

Ingredients:
- 2 cups mixed greens
- 1 cup cooked turkey breast, sliced
- 1/2 avocado, sliced
- 1/4 cup red onion, diced
- 2 tablespoons olive oil
- 1 tablespoon apple cider vinegar
- Sea salt and black pepper to taste

Instructions:
1. In a large bowl, combine mixed greens, sliced turkey, avocado slices, and red onion.
2. Drizzle with olive oil and apple cider vinegar.
3. Season with salt and pepper, then toss to combine.
4. Serve immediately.

Health Problems Addressed: Inflammation, nutrient deficiencies

Health Benefits: High in protein and healthy fats

Scientific Benefits: Turkey provides lean protein; avocado is rich in healthy fats

"This salad is creamy and delicious. It's a perfect lunch option that's both healthy and satisfying."

97. Shrimp and Mango Lettuce Wraps

Ingredients:
- 4 large lettuce leaves
- 1/2 cup cooked shrimp, peeled and deveined
- 1/2 mango, diced
- 1/4 cup red bell pepper, diced
- 1 tablespoon fresh lime juice
- Sea salt and black pepper to taste

Instructions:
1. Lay out lettuce leaves on a flat surface.
2. Divide cooked shrimp, diced mango, and red bell pepper evenly among the lettuce leaves.
3. Drizzle with fresh lime juice.
4. Season with salt and pepper.
5. Roll up the lettuce leaves to form wraps.
6. Serve immediately.

Health Problems Addressed: Inflammation, nutrient deficiencies

Health Benefits: High in protein, vitamins, and antioxidants

Scientific Benefits: Mango is rich in vitamins A and C; shrimp provides lean protein

"These lettuce wraps are tropical and delicious. They're a great lunch option that's both healthy and tasty."

98. Beef and Spinach Salad

Ingredients:
- 2 cups spinach leaves
- 1 cup cooked beef, sliced
- 1/4 cup cherry tomatoes, halved
- 1/4 cup red onion, diced
- 2 tablespoons olive oil
- 1 tablespoon balsamic vinegar
- Sea salt and black pepper to taste

Instructions:
1. In a large bowl, combine spinach leaves, sliced beef, cherry tomatoes, and red onion.
2. Drizzle with olive oil and balsamic vinegar.
3. Season with salt and pepper, then toss to combine.
4. Serve immediately.

Health Problems Addressed: Inflammation, nutrient deficiencies

Health Benefits: High in protein, vitamins, and antioxidants

Scientific Benefits: Spinach is rich in iron and magnesium; beef provides iron and protein

"This salad is hearty and flavorful. It's a great lunch that's both filling and nutritious."

99. Chicken and Strawberry Salad

Ingredients:
- 2 cups mixed greens
- 1 cup cooked chicken breast, sliced
- 1/2 cup strawberries, sliced
- 1/4 cup walnuts, chopped
- 2 tablespoons olive oil
- 1 tablespoon balsamic vinegar
- Sea salt and black pepper to taste

Instructions:
1. In a large bowl, combine mixed greens, sliced chicken, strawberries, and walnuts.
2. Drizzle with olive oil and balsamic vinegar.
3. Season with salt and pepper, then toss to combine.

4. Serve immediately.

Health Problems Addressed: Inflammation, nutrient deficiencies

Health Benefits: High in protein, vitamins, and antioxidants

Scientific Benefits: Strawberries are rich in vitamin C; chicken provides lean protein

"This salad is fresh and sweet. It's a delicious and healthy lunch option."

100. Tuna and Mango Salad

Ingredients:
- 2 cups mixed greens
- 2 cans tuna in water, drained
- 1/2 mango, diced
- 1/4 cup red onion, diced
- 2 tablespoons olive oil
- 1 tablespoon fresh lime juice
- Sea salt and black pepper to taste

Instructions:
1. In a large bowl, combine mixed greens, drained tuna, diced mango, and red onion.

2. Drizzle with olive oil and fresh lime juice.
3. Season with salt and pepper, then toss to combine.
4. Serve immediately.

Health Problems Addressed: Inflammation, nutrient deficiencies

Health Benefits: High in protein, omega-3 fatty acids, and vitamins

Scientific Benefits: Tuna provides lean protein and omega-3s; mango is rich in vitamins A and C

"This salad is light and tropical. It's a perfect lunch option that's both healthy and delicious."

These recipes are designed to provide a variety of flavors, textures, and nutrients while adhering to the principles of the Autoimmune Paleo Diet. Enjoy exploring these energizing lunches to support your health and wellness journey.

Chapter 4: Nourishing Dinners

101. Lemon Herb Roasted Chicken

Ingredients:
- 1 whole chicken
- 1/4 cup olive oil
- 2 lemons, sliced
- 4 garlic cloves, minced
- 1 tablespoon fresh rosemary, chopped
- 1 tablespoon fresh thyme, chopped
- Sea salt and black pepper to taste

Instructions:
1. Preheat the oven to 375°F (190°C).
2. In a bowl, mix olive oil, garlic, rosemary, thyme, salt, and pepper.
3. Rub the mixture all over the chicken and place lemon slices inside the cavity.
4. Roast in the oven for 1.5 to 2 hours, or until the internal temperature reaches 165°F (74°C).
5. Let rest for 10 minutes before carving.

Health Problems Addressed: Inflammation, nutrient deficiencies

Health Benefits: High in protein, antioxidants, and vitamins

Scientific Benefits: Herbs like rosemary and thyme have anti-inflammatory properties

"The aroma of this roasted chicken fills the house, making dinner time a special event."

102. Baked Cod with Asparagus

Ingredients:
- 4 cod fillets
- 1 bunch asparagus, trimmed
- 1 lemon, sliced
- 2 tablespoons olive oil
- 2 garlic cloves, minced
- Sea salt and black pepper to taste

Instructions:
1. Preheat the oven to 400°F (200°C).
2. Place cod fillets and asparagus on a baking sheet.
3. Drizzle with olive oil, and sprinkle with garlic, salt, and pepper.
4. Lay lemon slices on top of the cod.
5. Bake for 15-20 minutes, or until the cod is opaque and flakes easily.

Health Problems Addressed: Inflammation, nutrient deficiencies

Health Benefits: High in protein, omega-3 fatty acids, and vitamins

Scientific Benefits: Cod is a lean protein source; asparagus is rich in fiber and vitamins

 "This dish is light yet satisfying, perfect for a healthy and delicious dinner."

103. Beef and Vegetable Stir-Fry

Ingredients:
- 1 lb beef sirloin, thinly sliced
- 2 tablespoons coconut oil
- 1 bell pepper, sliced
- 1 zucchini, sliced
- 1 cup broccoli florets
- 2 garlic cloves, minced
- 2 tablespoons coconut aminos
- Sea salt and black pepper to taste

Instructions:
1. Heat coconut oil in a large skillet over medium-high heat.

2. Add beef and cook until browned. Remove from the skillet.
3. Add vegetables and cook until tender-crisp.
4. Return beef to the skillet and add garlic, coconut aminos, salt, and pepper.
5. Stir-fry for another 2-3 minutes.

Health Problems Addressed: Inflammation, nutrient deficiencies

Health Benefits: High in protein, vitamins, and antioxidants

Scientific Benefits: Broccoli is rich in vitamins C and K; beef provides iron and protein

"This stir-fry is quick, easy, and bursting with flavor. Perfect for busy weeknights."

104. Herb-Crusted Pork Tenderloin

Ingredients:
- 1 pork tenderloin
- 2 tablespoons olive oil
- 1 tablespoon fresh rosemary, chopped
- 1 tablespoon fresh thyme, chopped
- 2 garlic cloves, minced
- Sea salt and black pepper to taste

Instructions:

1. Preheat the oven to 375°F (190°C).
2. In a bowl, mix olive oil, rosemary, thyme, garlic, salt, and pepper.
3. Rub the mixture all over the pork tenderloin.
4. Place on a baking sheet and roast for 25-30 minutes, or until the internal temperature reaches 145°F (63°C).
5. Let rest for 10 minutes before slicing.

Health Problems Addressed: Inflammation, nutrient deficiencies

Health Benefits: High in protein, antioxidants, and vitamins

Scientific Benefits: Pork is a good source of lean protein; herbs provide anti-inflammatory benefits

"This tenderloin is juicy and full of herbaceous flavor. It's a hit with the whole family."

105. Sweet Potato and Kale Curry

Ingredients:
- 1 tablespoon coconut oil
- 1 onion, diced
- 2 garlic cloves, minced

- 1 tablespoon fresh ginger, minced
- 2 sweet potatoes, peeled and cubed
- 1 can coconut milk
- 2 cups vegetable broth
- 2 cups kale, chopped
- 2 tablespoons curry powder
- Sea salt and black pepper to taste

Instructions:
1. Heat coconut oil in a large pot over medium heat.
2. Add onion, garlic, and ginger, and cook until fragrant.
3. Add sweet potatoes, coconut milk, vegetable broth, and curry powder.
4. Bring to a simmer and cook until sweet potatoes are tender.
5. Stir in kale and cook until wilted.
6. Season with salt and pepper before serving.

Health Problems Addressed: Inflammation, nutrient deficiencies

Health Benefits: High in vitamins, fiber, and antioxidants

Scientific Benefits: Sweet potatoes are rich in vitamins A and C; kale is nutrient-dense and anti-inflammatory

"This curry is comforting and packed with flavor. It's a great way to incorporate more vegetables into dinner."

106. Lemon Garlic Shrimp

Ingredients:
- 1 lb large shrimp, peeled and deveined
- 2 tablespoons olive oil
- 4 garlic cloves, minced
- 1 lemon, juiced and zested
- 1/4 cup fresh parsley, chopped
- Sea salt and black pepper to taste

Instructions:
1. Heat olive oil in a large skillet over medium heat.
2. Add garlic and cook until fragrant.
3. Add shrimp and cook until pink and opaque.
4. Stir in lemon juice, zest, parsley, salt, and pepper.
5. Serve immediately.

Health Problems Addressed: Inflammation, nutrient deficiencies

Health Benefits: High in protein, omega-3 fatty acids, and antioxidants

Scientific Benefits: Shrimp is a lean protein source; garlic and lemon provide antioxidants and anti-inflammatory benefits

"These shrimp are zesty and delicious. Perfect for a quick and healthy dinner."

107. Chicken and Broccoli Casserole

Ingredients:
- 2 tablespoons coconut oil
- 1 onion, diced
- 2 garlic cloves, minced
- 2 cups cooked chicken breast, shredded
- 4 cups broccoli florets
- 1 can coconut milk
- 1/2 cup chicken broth
- Sea salt and black pepper to taste

Instructions:
1. Preheat the oven to 375°F (190°C).
2. Heat coconut oil in a skillet over medium heat. Add onion and cook until translucent.
3. Add garlic and cook for 1-2 minutes.
4. In a large bowl, combine shredded chicken, broccoli, coconut milk, chicken broth, salt, and pepper.
5. Transfer mixture to a baking dish.
6. Bake for 25-30 minutes until the top is golden and bubbly.

Health Problems Addressed: Inflammation, nutrient deficiencies

Health Benefits: High in protein, vitamins, and antioxidants

Scientific Benefits: Broccoli is rich in vitamins C and K; chicken provides lean protein

"This casserole is creamy and comforting. It's a family favorite for busy weeknights."

108. Balsamic Glazed Steak

Ingredients:
- 2 steaks (your choice of cut)
- 1/4 cup balsamic vinegar
- 2 tablespoons olive oil
- 2 garlic cloves, minced
- 1 tablespoon fresh rosemary, chopped
- Sea salt and black pepper to taste

Instructions:
1. In a bowl, mix balsamic vinegar, olive oil, garlic, rosemary, salt, and pepper.
2. Marinate the steaks in the mixture for at least 30 minutes.
3. Preheat a grill or skillet over medium-high heat.
4. Cook steaks to desired doneness, basting with the marinade.

5. Let rest for 5 minutes before serving.

Health Problems Addressed: Inflammation, nutrient deficiencies

Health Benefits: High in protein and antioxidants

Scientific Benefits: Beef provides iron and protein; balsamic vinegar has antioxidant properties

"This steak is flavorful and juicy. The balsamic glaze adds a delicious tang."

109. Stuffed Bell Peppers

Ingredients:
- 4 bell peppers, tops cut off and seeds removed
- 1 lb ground turkey
- 1 onion, diced
- 2 garlic cloves, minced
- 1 zucchini, diced
- 1 cup spinach, chopped
- 1 can diced tomatoes
- Sea salt and black pepper to taste

Instructions:
1. Preheat the oven to 375°F (190°C).

2. Heat a skillet over medium heat and cook ground turkey until browned.

3. Add onion, garlic, zucchini, and spinach, and cook until vegetables are tender.

4. Stir in diced tomatoes, salt, and pepper.

5. Stuff the mixture into bell peppers and place in a baking dish.

6. Bake for 25-30 minutes until peppers are tender.

Health Problems Addressed: Inflammation, nutrient deficiencies

Health Benefits: High in protein, vitamins, and antioxidants

Scientific Benefits: Bell peppers are rich in vitamins A and C; turkey provides lean protein

"These stuffed peppers are hearty and packed with flavor. A great way to enjoy a balanced meal."

110. Ginger Sesame Chicken

Ingredients:
- 1 lb chicken breast, thinly sliced
- 2 tablespoons coconut oil
- 2 tablespoons fresh ginger, minced
- 2 garlic cloves, minced

- 2 tablespoons coconut aminos
- 1 tablespoon sesame oil
- 1 tablespoon sesame seeds
- 1 green onion, sliced
- Sea salt and black pepper to taste

Instructions:
1. Heat coconut oil in a skillet over medium heat.
2. Add ginger and garlic, and cook until fragrant.
3. Add chicken and cook until browned.
4. Stir in coconut aminos, sesame oil, sesame seeds, salt, and pepper.
5. Cook for another 2-3 minutes.
6. Garnish with green onion before serving.

Health Problems Addressed: Inflammation, nutrient deficiencies

Health Benefits: High in protein, antioxidants, and healthy fats

Scientific Benefits: Ginger and garlic have anti-inflammatory properties; chicken provides lean protein

"This chicken is savory and delicious. The ginger and sesame add a wonderful depth of flavor."

111. Garlic and Herb Lamb Chops

Ingredients:
- 4 lamb chops
- 2 tablespoons olive oil
- 4 garlic cloves, minced
- 1 tablespoon fresh rosemary, chopped
- 1 tablespoon fresh thyme, chopped
- Sea salt and black pepper to taste

Instructions:
1. Preheat grill or skillet to medium-high heat.
2. In a bowl, mix olive oil, garlic, rosemary, thyme, salt, and pepper.
3. Rub the mixture all over the lamb chops.
4. Grill or pan-fry lamb chops for 3-4 minutes per side for medium-rare.
5. Let rest for 5 minutes before serving.

Health Problems Addressed: Inflammation, nutrient deficiencies

Health Benefits: High in protein, healthy fats, and antioxidants

Scientific Benefits: Lamb is rich in protein and iron; herbs have anti-inflammatory benefits

"These lamb chops are tender and flavorful. A perfect dinner for special occasions."

112. Cauliflower and Beef Shepherd's Pie

Ingredients:
- 1 lb ground beef
- 1 onion, diced
- 2 garlic cloves, minced
- 2 carrots, diced
- 1 cup green peas
- 1 head cauliflower, chopped
- 1/4 cup coconut milk
- 2 tablespoons olive oil
- Sea salt and black pepper to taste

Instructions:
1. Preheat the oven to 375°F (190°C).
2. Heat a skillet over medium heat and cook ground beef until browned.
3. Add onion, garlic, carrots, and peas, and cook until vegetables are tender. Season with salt and pepper.
4. Steam cauliflower until tender. Mash with coconut milk, olive oil, salt, and pepper.
5. Transfer beef mixture to a baking dish and top with mashed cauliflower.
6. Bake for 20-25 minutes until golden and bubbly.

Health Problems Addressed: Inflammation, nutrient deficiencies

Health Benefits: High in protein, vitamins, and fiber

Scientific Benefits: Cauliflower is rich in fiber and antioxidants; beef provides iron and protein

"This shepherd's pie is comforting and hearty. The cauliflower mash is a great alternative to potatoes."

113. Lemon Dill Salmon

Ingredients:
- 4 salmon fillets
- 2 tablespoons olive oil
- 1 lemon, sliced
- 1/4 cup fresh dill, chopped
- Sea salt and black pepper to taste

Instructions:
1. Preheat the oven to 375°F (190°C).
2. Place salmon fillets on a baking sheet and drizzle with olive oil.
3. Top with lemon slices, fresh dill, salt, and pepper.
4. Bake for 15-20 minutes, or until salmon is cooked through.
5. Serve immediately.

Health Problems Addressed: Inflammation, nutrient deficiencies

Health Benefits: High in protein, omega-3 fatty acids, and antioxidants

Scientific Benefits: Salmon is rich in omega-3s; dill has antioxidant properties

"This salmon is light and flavorful. The lemon and dill complement the fish perfectly."

114. Turkey and Zucchini Meatballs

Ingredients:
- 1 lb ground turkey
- 1 zucchini, grated
- 1/4 cup fresh parsley, chopped
- 2 garlic cloves, minced
- 1 egg
- Sea salt and black pepper to taste

Instructions:
1. Preheat the oven to 375°F (190°C).
2. In a large bowl, combine ground turkey, grated zucchini, parsley, garlic, egg, salt, and pepper.

3. Form mixture into meatballs and place on a baking sheet.
4. Bake for 20-25 minutes, or until cooked through.
5. Serve with your favorite AIP-friendly sauce.

Health Problems Addressed: Inflammation, nutrient deficiencies

Health Benefits: High in protein and vitamins

Scientific Benefits: Turkey is a lean protein source; zucchini adds moisture and nutrients

"These meatballs are juicy and delicious. A great way to sneak in some extra vegetables."

115. Garlic Shrimp and Cauliflower Rice

Ingredients:
- 1 lb large shrimp, peeled and deveined
- 2 tablespoons coconut oil
- 4 garlic cloves, minced
- 1 head cauliflower, grated (to make rice)
- 1/4 cup fresh parsley, chopped
- Sea salt and black pepper to taste

Instructions:
1. Heat coconut oil in a large skillet over medium heat.

2. Add garlic and cook until fragrant.

3. Add shrimp and cook until pink and opaque. Remove shrimp from the skillet.

4. Add grated cauliflower to the skillet and cook until tender.

5. Stir in fresh parsley, salt, and pepper.

6. Return shrimp to the skillet and toss to combine.

7. Serve immediately.

Health Problems Addressed: Inflammation, nutrient deficiencies

Health Benefits: High in protein, fiber, and antioxidants

Scientific Benefits: Cauliflower is rich in fiber and vitamins; shrimp provides lean protein

"This dish is light and satisfying. The cauliflower rice is a great low-carb alternative."

116. Herb Roasted Pork Chops

Ingredients:
- 4 pork chops
- 2 tablespoons olive oil
- 2 garlic cloves, minced
- 1 tablespoon fresh rosemary, chopped
- 1 tablespoon fresh thyme, chopped

- Sea salt and black pepper to taste

Instructions:
1. Preheat the oven to 375°F (190°C).
2. In a bowl, mix olive oil, garlic, rosemary, thyme, salt, and pepper.
3. Rub the mixture all over the pork chops.
4. Place on a baking sheet and roast for 20-25 minutes, or until the internal temperature reaches 145°F (63°C).
5. Let rest for 5 minutes before serving.

Health Problems Addressed: Inflammation, nutrient deficiencies

Health Benefits: High in protein, antioxidants, and vitamins

Scientific Benefits: Pork is a good source of lean protein; herbs provide anti-inflammatory benefits

"These pork chops are flavorful and juicy. The herb rub adds a delicious touch."

117. Chicken and Vegetable Skewers

Ingredients:
- 1 lb chicken breast, cubed
- 1 bell pepper, cubed

- 1 zucchini, sliced
- 1 red onion, cubed
- 2 tablespoons olive oil
- 1 tablespoon fresh thyme, chopped
- Sea salt and black pepper to taste

Instructions:
1. Preheat the grill to medium-high heat.
2. In a bowl, mix olive oil, thyme, salt, and pepper.
3. Thread chicken and vegetables onto skewers and brush with the olive oil mixture.
4. Grill for 10-12 minutes, turning occasionally, until chicken is cooked through.
5. Serve immediately.

Health Problems Addressed: Inflammation, nutrient deficiencies

Health Benefits: High in protein, vitamins, and antioxidants

Scientific Benefits: Bell peppers are rich in vitamins A and C; chicken provides lean protein

"These skewers are colorful and delicious. Perfect for a summer barbecue."

118. Baked Salmon with Dill and Lemon

Ingredients:
- 4 salmon fillets
- 2 tablespoons olive oil
- 1 lemon, sliced
- 1/4 cup fresh dill, chopped
- Sea salt and black pepper to taste

Instructions:
1. Preheat the oven to 375°F (190°C).
2. Place salmon fillets on a baking sheet and drizzle with olive oil.
3. Top with lemon slices, fresh dill, salt, and pepper.
4. Bake for 15-20 minutes, or until salmon is cooked through.
5. Serve immediately.

Health Problems Addressed: Inflammation, nutrient deficiencies

Health Benefits: High in protein, omega-3 fatty acids, and antioxidants

Scientific Benefits: Salmon is rich in omega-3s; dill has antioxidant properties

"This salmon is light and flavorful. The lemon and dill complement the fish perfectly."

119. Sweet Potato and Beef Stew

Ingredients:
- 1 lb beef stew meat
- 2 tablespoons coconut oil
- 1 onion, diced
- 2 garlic cloves, minced
- 2 sweet potatoes, peeled and cubed
- 4 cups beef broth
- 2 carrots, sliced
- Sea salt and black pepper to taste

Instructions:
1. Heat coconut oil in a large pot over medium heat.
2. Add beef and brown on all sides.
3. Add onion, garlic, sweet potatoes, beef broth, carrots, salt, and pepper.
4. Bring to a simmer and cook for 1-2 hours, or until beef is tender.
5. Serve hot.

Health Problems Addressed: Inflammation, nutrient deficiencies

Health Benefits: High in protein, vitamins, and fiber

Scientific Benefits: Sweet potatoes are rich in vitamins A and C; beef provides iron and protein

"This stew is hearty and comforting. Perfect for a cold winter night."

120. Lemon Herb Chicken Thighs

Ingredients:
- 4 chicken thighs
- 2 tablespoons olive oil
- 1 lemon, juiced and zested
- 2 garlic cloves, minced
- 1 tablespoon fresh thyme, chopped
- Sea salt and black pepper to taste

Instructions:
1. Preheat the oven to 375°F (190°C).
2. In a bowl, mix olive oil, lemon juice, zest, garlic, thyme, salt, and pepper.
3. Rub the mixture all over the chicken thighs.
4. Place on a baking sheet and roast for 25-30 minutes, or until the internal temperature reaches 165°F (74°C).
5. Let rest for 5 minutes before serving.

Health Problems Addressed: Inflammation, nutrient deficiencies

Health Benefits: High in protein, antioxidants, and vitamins

Scientific Benefits: Chicken thighs are rich in protein and iron; lemon and herbs provide antioxidants

"These chicken thighs are juicy and flavorful. The lemon and herbs add a bright, fresh taste."

121. Garlic and Herb Baked Chicken

Ingredients:
- 4 chicken breasts
- 2 tablespoons olive oil
- 4 garlic cloves, minced
- 1 tablespoon fresh rosemary, chopped
- 1 tablespoon fresh thyme, chopped
- Sea salt and black pepper to taste

Instructions:
1. Preheat the oven to 375°F (190°C).
2. In a bowl, mix olive oil, garlic, rosemary, thyme, salt, and pepper.
3. Rub the mixture all over the chicken breasts.
4. Place on a baking sheet and bake for 25-30 minutes, or until the internal temperature reaches 165°F (74°C).
5. Let rest for 5 minutes before serving.

Health Problems Addressed: Inflammation, nutrient deficiencies

Health Benefits: High in protein, antioxidants, and vitamins

Scientific Benefits: Chicken breasts are a lean protein source; garlic and herbs provide anti-inflammatory benefits

"This baked chicken is simple yet delicious. Perfect for a quick and healthy dinner."

122. Beef and Cabbage Stir-Fry

Ingredients:
- 1 lb ground beef
- 2 tablespoons coconut oil
- 1 onion, diced
- 2 garlic cloves, minced
- 4 cups shredded cabbage
- 2 tablespoons coconut aminos
- Sea salt and black pepper to taste

Instructions:
1. Heat coconut oil in a large skillet over medium heat.
2. Add ground beef and cook until browned.

3. Add onion, garlic, and cabbage, and cook until vegetables are tender.

4. Stir in coconut aminos, salt, and pepper.

5. Cook for another 2-3 minutes.

Health Problems Addressed: Inflammation, nutrient deficiencies

Health Benefits: High in protein, vitamins, and antioxidants

Scientific Benefits: Cabbage is rich in vitamins C and K; beef provides iron and protein

"This stir-fry is quick, easy, and delicious. Perfect for a busy weeknight dinner."

123. Herb-Crusted Salmon

Ingredients:
- 4 salmon fillets
- 2 tablespoons olive oil
- 1/4 cup fresh parsley, chopped
- 1 tablespoon fresh dill, chopped
- 1 tablespoon fresh thyme, chopped
- Sea salt and black pepper to taste

Instructions:

1. Preheat the oven to 375°F (190°C).
2. In a bowl, mix olive oil, parsley, dill, thyme, salt, and pepper.
3. Rub the mixture all over the salmon fillets.
4. Place on a baking sheet and bake for 15-20 minutes, or until the salmon is cooked through.
5. Serve immediately.

Health Problems Addressed: Inflammation, nutrient deficiencies

Health Benefits: High in protein, omega-3 fatty acids, and antioxidants

Scientific Benefits: Salmon is rich in omega-3s; herbs have anti-inflammatory properties

"This salmon is flavorful and healthy. The herb crust adds a wonderful texture."

124. Balsamic Chicken and Vegetables

Ingredients:
- 4 chicken breasts
- 2 tablespoons olive oil
- 1/4 cup balsamic vinegar
- 1 bell pepper, sliced
- 1 zucchini, sliced

- 1 red onion, sliced
- Sea salt and black pepper to taste

Instructions:
1. Preheat the oven to 375°F (190°C).
2. In a bowl, mix olive oil, balsamic vinegar, salt, and pepper.
3. Place chicken breasts and vegetables on a baking sheet.
4. Drizzle with the balsamic mixture.
5. Bake for 25-30 minutes, or until the chicken is cooked through and vegetables are tender.

Health Problems Addressed: Inflammation, nutrient deficiencies

Health Benefits: High in protein, vitamins, and antioxidants

Scientific Benefits: Balsamic vinegar has antioxidant properties; chicken provides lean protein

"This dish is colorful and flavorful. The balsamic vinegar adds a delicious tang."

125. Lemon Garlic Tilapia

Ingredients:

- 4 tilapia fillets
- 2 tablespoons olive oil
- 4 garlic cloves, minced
- 1 lemon, juiced and zested
- Sea salt and black pepper to taste

Instructions:
1. Preheat the oven to 375°F (190°C).
2. Place tilapia fillets on a baking sheet and drizzle with olive oil.
3. Top with garlic, lemon juice, zest, salt, and pepper.
4. Bake for 15-20 minutes, or until the tilapia is cooked through.
5. Serve immediately.

Health Problems Addressed: Inflammation, nutrient deficiencies

Health Benefits: High in protein and omega-3 fatty acids

Scientific Benefits: Tilapia is a lean protein source; lemon and garlic provide antioxidants and anti-inflammatory benefits

"This tilapia is light and zesty. Perfect for a quick and healthy dinner."

126. Stuffed Acorn Squash

Ingredients:
- 2 acorn squashes, halved and seeds removed
- 1 lb ground turkey
- 1 onion, diced
- 2 garlic cloves, minced
- 1 apple, diced
- 1/4 cup fresh parsley, chopped
- Sea salt and black pepper to taste

Instructions:
1. Preheat the oven to 375°F (190°C).
2. Place acorn squash halves on a baking sheet and bake for 25-30 minutes, or until tender.
3. Heat a skillet over medium heat and cook ground turkey until browned.
4. Add onion, garlic, and apple, and cook until tender.
5. Stir in fresh parsley, salt, and pepper.
6. Stuff the mixture into the baked acorn squash halves and serve.

Health Problems Addressed: Inflammation, nutrient deficiencies

Health Benefits: High in protein, vitamins, and fiber

Scientific Benefits: Acorn squash is rich in vitamins A and C; turkey provides lean protein

"These stuffed squashes are hearty and delicious. A great fall dinner option."

127. Ginger Lime Chicken Thighs

Ingredients:
- 4 chicken thighs
- 2 tablespoons olive oil
- 2 tablespoons fresh ginger, minced
- 1 lime, juiced and zested
- Sea salt and black pepper to taste

Instructions:
1. Preheat the oven to 375°F (190°C).
2. In a bowl, mix olive oil, ginger, lime juice, zest, salt, and pepper.
3. Rub the mixture all over the chicken thighs.
4. Place on a baking sheet and roast for 25-30 minutes, or until the internal temperature reaches 165°F (74°C).
5. Let rest for 5 minutes before serving.

Health Problems Addressed: Inflammation, nutrient deficiencies

Health Benefits: High in protein, antioxidants, and vitamins

Scientific Benefits: Chicken thighs are rich in protein and iron; ginger and lime have anti-inflammatory benefits

"These chicken thighs are tangy and flavorful. The ginger and lime add a refreshing kick."

128. Baked Cod with Tomato and Basil

Ingredients:
- 4 cod fillets
- 2 tablespoons olive oil
- 1 cup cherry tomatoes, halved
- 1/4 cup fresh basil, chopped
- 2 garlic cloves, minced
- Sea salt and black pepper to taste

Instructions:
1. Preheat the oven to 375°F (190°C).
2. Place cod fillets on a baking sheet and drizzle with olive oil.
3. Top with cherry tomatoes, fresh basil, garlic, salt, and pepper.
4. Bake for 15-20 minutes, or until the cod is cooked through.
5. Serve immediately.

Health Problems Addressed: Inflammation, nutrient deficiencies

Health Benefits: High in protein, omega-3 fatty acids, and antioxidants

Scientific Benefits: Cod is a lean protein source; tomatoes and basil provide antioxidants

"This cod is light and fresh. The tomatoes and basil add a burst of flavor."

129. Spinach and Artichoke Chicken

Ingredients:
- 4 chicken breasts
- 2 tablespoons olive oil
- 2 garlic cloves, minced
- 1 cup spinach, chopped
- 1 cup artichoke hearts, chopped
- Sea salt and black pepper to taste

Instructions:
1. Preheat the oven to 375°F (190°C).
2. Heat olive oil in a skillet over medium heat.
3. Add garlic and cook until fragrant.
4. Stir in spinach and artichokes, and cook until spinach is wilted.

5. Season with salt and pepper.
6. Place chicken breasts on a baking sheet and top with the spinach and artichoke mixture.
7. Bake for 25-30 minutes, or until the chicken is cooked through.

Health Problems Addressed: Inflammation, nutrient deficiencies

Health Benefits: High in protein, vitamins, and antioxidants

Scientific Benefits: Spinach is rich in vitamins A and C; chicken provides lean protein

"This chicken is delicious and packed with nutrients. The spinach and artichokes add a nice texture."

130. Lemon Basil Chicken

Ingredients:
- 4 chicken breasts
- 2 tablespoons olive oil
- 1 lemon, juiced and zested
- 1/4 cup fresh basil, chopped
- Sea salt and black pepper to taste

Instructions:

1. Preheat the oven to 375°F (190°C).
2. In a bowl, mix olive oil, lemon juice, zest, basil, salt, and pepper.
3. Rub the mixture all over the chicken breasts.
4. Place on a baking sheet and bake for 25-30 minutes, or until the internal temperature reaches 165°F (74°C).
5. Let rest for 5 minutes before serving.

Health Problems Addressed: Inflammation, nutrient deficiencies

Health Benefits: High in protein, antioxidants, and vitamins

Scientific Benefits: Chicken breasts are a lean protein source; lemon and basil provide antioxidants

"This chicken is light and flavorful. The lemon and basil add a refreshing taste."

131. Spaghetti Squash with Pesto Chicken

Ingredients:
- 1 large spaghetti squash
- 2 tablespoons olive oil
- 1 lb chicken breast, cubed
- 1/2 cup fresh basil, chopped
- 1/4 cup pine nuts

- 2 garlic cloves
- 1/4 cup olive oil
- Sea salt and black pepper to taste

Instructions:
1. Preheat the oven to 375°F (190°C). Cut the spaghetti squash in half, remove seeds, and brush with olive oil. Bake cut side down for 30-40 minutes.
2. While the squash bakes, prepare the pesto by blending basil, pine nuts, garlic, olive oil, salt, and pepper until smooth.
3. Heat a skillet over medium heat and cook chicken until browned.
4. Once the squash is cooked, use a fork to scrape out the strands. Mix the spaghetti squash with pesto and top with the chicken.

Health Problems Addressed: Inflammation, nutrient deficiencies

Health Benefits: High in protein, vitamins, and healthy fats

Scientific Benefits: Basil and pine nuts are rich in antioxidants; chicken provides lean protein

"This dish is incredibly satisfying. The spaghetti squash is a great pasta substitute, and the pesto is fresh and vibrant."

132. Lemon Rosemary Pork Tenderloin

Ingredients:
- 1 pork tenderloin
- 2 tablespoons olive oil
- 2 garlic cloves, minced
- 1 lemon, juiced and zested
- 2 tablespoons fresh rosemary, chopped
- Sea salt and black pepper to taste

Instructions:
1. Preheat the oven to 400°F (200°C).
2. Mix olive oil, garlic, lemon juice, zest, rosemary, salt, and pepper. Rub the mixture over the pork tenderloin.
3. Place tenderloin in a baking dish and roast for 25-30 minutes, or until the internal temperature reaches 145°F (63°C).
4. Let rest for 5 minutes before slicing and serving.

Health Problems Addressed: Inflammation, nutrient deficiencies

Health Benefits: High in protein, antioxidants, and healthy fats

Scientific Benefits: Pork is a good source of lean protein;
rosemary has anti-inflammatory properties

"The pork tenderloin is tender and juicy with a delicious
lemon rosemary flavor. Perfect for a family dinner."

133. Ginger Beef Stir-Fry

Ingredients:
- 1 lb beef sirloin, thinly sliced
- 2 tablespoons coconut oil
- 2 tablespoons fresh ginger, minced
- 3 garlic cloves, minced
- 1 bell pepper, sliced
- 1 cup broccoli florets
- 2 tablespoons coconut aminos
- Sea salt and black pepper to taste

Instructions:
1. Heat coconut oil in a large skillet over medium-high
heat.
2. Add ginger and garlic, and cook until fragrant.
3. Add beef and cook until browned.
4. Add bell pepper, broccoli, coconut aminos, salt, and
pepper. Cook until vegetables are tender.
5. Serve immediately.

Health Problems Addressed: Inflammation, nutrient deficiencies

Health Benefits: High in protein, vitamins, and antioxidants

Scientific Benefits: Broccoli is rich in vitamins C and K; beef provides iron and protein

"This stir-fry is quick, easy, and full of flavor. The ginger adds a nice kick."

134. Herb-Crusted Cod

Ingredients:
- 4 cod fillets
- 2 tablespoons olive oil
- 1/4 cup almond flour
- 1 tablespoon fresh parsley, chopped
- 1 tablespoon fresh thyme, chopped
- Sea salt and black pepper to taste

Instructions:
1. Preheat the oven to 375°F (190°C).
2. In a bowl, mix almond flour, parsley, thyme, salt, and pepper.
3. Brush cod fillets with olive oil and press into the herb mixture.

4. Place on a baking sheet and bake for 15-20 minutes, or until the fish is cooked through.

5. Serve immediately.

Health Problems Addressed: Inflammation, nutrient deficiencies

Health Benefits: High in protein, omega-3 fatty acids, and antioxidants

Scientific Benefits: Cod is a lean protein source; herbs provide anti-inflammatory benefits

"The cod is light and flaky with a delicious herb crust. Perfect for a healthy dinner."

135. Baked Lemon Garlic Shrimp

Ingredients:
- 1 lb large shrimp, peeled and deveined
- 2 tablespoons olive oil
- 4 garlic cloves, minced
- 1 lemon, juiced and zested
- Sea salt and black pepper to taste

Instructions:
1. Preheat the oven to 375°F (190°C).

2. In a bowl, mix olive oil, garlic, lemon juice, zest, salt, and pepper.
3. Toss shrimp in the mixture and place on a baking sheet.
4. Bake for 10-12 minutes, or until shrimp are pink and cooked through.
5. Serve immediately.

Health Problems Addressed: Inflammation, nutrient deficiencies

Health Benefits: High in protein, omega-3 fatty acids, and antioxidants

Scientific Benefits: Shrimp is a lean protein source; lemon and garlic provide anti-inflammatory benefits

"These shrimp are quick to make and incredibly flavorful. The lemon and garlic are a perfect pairing."

136. Spinach and Artichoke Stuffed Chicken

Ingredients:
- 4 chicken breasts
- 2 tablespoons olive oil
- 2 garlic cloves, minced
- 1 cup spinach, chopped
- 1/2 cup artichoke hearts, chopped

- Sea salt and black pepper to taste

Instructions:
1. Preheat the oven to 375°F (190°C).
2. Heat olive oil in a skillet over medium heat. Add garlic, spinach, and artichokes, and cook until spinach is wilted.
3. Cut a pocket in each chicken breast and stuff with the spinach and artichoke mixture. Secure with toothpicks.
4. Place chicken breasts on a baking sheet and bake for 25-30 minutes, or until cooked through.
5. Serve immediately.

Health Problems Addressed: Inflammation, nutrient deficiencies

Health Benefits: High in protein, vitamins, and antioxidants

Scientific Benefits: Spinach is rich in vitamins A and C; chicken provides lean protein

"This stuffed chicken is moist and flavorful. The spinach and artichoke filling is a delightful surprise."

137. Herb-Marinated Lamb Chops

Ingredients:

- 4 lamb chops
- 2 tablespoons olive oil
- 2 garlic cloves, minced
- 1 tablespoon fresh rosemary, chopped
- 1 tablespoon fresh thyme, chopped
- Sea salt and black pepper to taste

Instructions:

1. In a bowl, mix olive oil, garlic, rosemary, thyme, salt, and pepper. Rub the mixture over the lamb chops.
2. Preheat grill or skillet to medium-high heat.
3. Cook lamb chops for 3-4 minutes per side for medium-rare, or until desired doneness.
4. Let rest for 5 minutes before serving.

Health Problems Addressed: Inflammation, nutrient deficiencies

Health Benefits: High in protein, healthy fats, and antioxidants

Scientific Benefits: Lamb is rich in protein and iron; herbs provide anti-inflammatory benefits

"These lamb chops are tender and packed with flavor. Perfect for a special dinner."

138. Ginger Turmeric Chicken

Ingredients:
- 4 chicken thighs
- 2 tablespoons olive oil
- 2 tablespoons fresh ginger, minced
- 1 teaspoon ground turmeric
- Sea salt and black pepper to taste

Instructions:
1. Preheat the oven to 375°F (190°C).
2. In a bowl, mix olive oil, ginger, turmeric, salt, and pepper. Rub the mixture over the chicken thighs.
3. Place chicken thighs on a baking sheet and roast for 25-30 minutes, or until the internal temperature reaches 165°F (74°C).
4. Let rest for 5 minutes before serving.

Health Problems Addressed: Inflammation, nutrient deficiencies

Health Benefits: High in protein, antioxidants, and vitamins

Scientific Benefits: Chicken thighs are rich in protein and iron; ginger and turmeric have anti-inflammatory properties

"These chicken thighs are flavorful and healthy. The ginger and turmeric add a unique taste."

139. Coconut Curry Shrimp

Ingredients:
- 1 lb large shrimp, peeled and deveined
- 2 tablespoons coconut oil
- 1 onion, diced
- 2 garlic cloves, minced
- 1 tablespoon fresh ginger, minced
- 1 can (14 oz) coconut milk
- 2 tablespoons red curry paste
- 1 cup spinach, chopped
- Sea salt and black pepper to taste

Instructions:
1. Heat coconut oil in a large skillet over medium heat.
2. Add onion, garlic, and ginger, and cook until fragrant.
3. Stir in coconut milk and red curry paste, and bring to a simmer.
4. Add shrimp and spinach, and cook until shrimp are pink and cooked through.
5. Season with salt and pepper, and serve immediately.

Health Problems Addressed: Inflammation, nutrient deficiencies

Health Benefits: High in protein, healthy fats, and antioxidants

Scientific Benefits: Coconut milk is rich in healthy fats; shrimp provides lean protein

"This curry is creamy and delicious. The flavors are rich and comforting."

140. Roasted Garlic Herb Chicken

Ingredients:
- 1 whole chicken
- 4 tablespoons olive oil
- 6 garlic cloves, minced
- 1 tablespoon fresh rosemary, chopped
- 1 tablespoon fresh thyme, chopped
- Sea salt and black pepper to taste

Instructions:
1. Preheat the oven to 400°F (200°C).
2. In a bowl, mix olive oil, garlic, rosemary, thyme, salt, and pepper.
3. Rub the mixture all over the chicken.
4. Place chicken in a roasting pan and roast for 1-1.5 hours, or until the internal temperature reaches 165°F (74°C).
5. Let rest for 10 minutes before carving and serving.

Health Problems Addressed: Inflammation, nutrient deficiencies

Health Benefits: High in protein, antioxidants, and vitamins

Scientific Benefits: Chicken is a lean protein source; garlic and herbs provide anti-inflammatory benefits

"This roasted chicken is juicy and flavorful. The garlic and herbs make it incredibly aromatic."

141. Zucchini Noodles with Meatballs

Ingredients:
- 2 zucchinis, spiralized
- 1 lb ground beef
- 1 egg
- 1/4 cup almond flour
- 2 garlic cloves, minced
- 1/4 cup fresh parsley, chopped
- 2 tablespoons olive oil
- 2 cups marinara sauce (AIP-friendly)
- Sea salt and black pepper to taste

Instructions:
1. Preheat the oven to 375°F (190°C).

2. In a bowl, mix ground beef, egg, almond flour, garlic, parsley, salt, and pepper. Form into meatballs.

3. Place meatballs on a baking sheet and bake for 20-25 minutes, or until cooked through.

4. Heat olive oil in a skillet and sauté zucchini noodles until tender.

5. Serve meatballs over zucchini noodles with marinara sauce.

Health Problems Addressed: Inflammation, nutrient deficiencies

Health Benefits: High in protein, vitamins, and antioxidants

Scientific Benefits: Zucchini is low in calories and rich in vitamins; beef provides iron and protein

"This dish is a great pasta alternative. The meatballs are flavorful and the zucchini noodles are light and refreshing."

142. Lemon Dill Baked Salmon

Ingredients:
- 4 salmon fillets
- 2 tablespoons olive oil
- 1 lemon, sliced

- 1/4 cup fresh dill, chopped
- Sea salt and black pepper to taste

Instructions:
1. Preheat the oven to 375°F (190°C).
2. Place salmon fillets on a baking sheet and drizzle with olive oil.
3. Top with lemon slices, dill, salt, and pepper.
4. Bake for 15-20 minutes, or until the salmon is cooked through.
5. Serve immediately.

Health Problems Addressed: Inflammation, nutrient deficiencies

Health Benefits: High in protein, omega-3 fatty acids, and antioxidants

Scientific Benefits: Salmon is rich in omega-3s; dill has anti-inflammatory properties

"This salmon is light and fresh. The lemon and dill add a wonderful flavor."

143. Butternut Squash and Sage Chicken

Ingredients:
- 4 chicken thighs

- 2 tablespoons olive oil
- 1 butternut squash, peeled and cubed
- 1 tablespoon fresh sage, chopped
- Sea salt and black pepper to taste

Instructions:
1. Preheat the oven to 375°F (190°C).
2. Place chicken thighs and butternut squash on a baking sheet.
3. Drizzle with olive oil and sprinkle with sage, salt, and pepper.
4. Bake for 25-30 minutes, or until the chicken is cooked through and squash is tender.
5. Serve immediately.

Health Problems Addressed: Inflammation, nutrient deficiencies

Health Benefits: High in protein, vitamins, and antioxidants

Scientific Benefits: Butternut squash is rich in vitamins A and C; chicken provides lean protein

"This dish is hearty and satisfying. The butternut squash and sage pair perfectly with the chicken."

144. Basil Pesto Chicken

Ingredients:
- 4 chicken breasts
- 2 tablespoons olive oil
- 1/2 cup fresh basil, chopped
- 1/4 cup pine nuts
- 2 garlic cloves
- Sea salt and black pepper to taste

Instructions:
1. Preheat the oven to 375°F (190°C).
2. In a food processor, blend basil, pine nuts, garlic, olive oil, salt, and pepper until smooth.
3. Rub the pesto over the chicken breasts.
4. Place on a baking sheet and bake for 25-30 minutes, or until the internal temperature reaches 165°F (74°C).
5. Let rest for 5 minutes before serving.

Health Problems Addressed: Inflammation, nutrient deficiencies

Health Benefits: High in protein, healthy fats, and antioxidants

Scientific Benefits: Basil and pine nuts are rich in antioxidants; chicken provides lean protein

"This chicken is bursting with flavor. The basil pesto is fresh and vibrant."

145. Coconut Lime Shrimp

Ingredients:
- 1 lb large shrimp, peeled and deveined
- 2 tablespoons coconut oil
- 1 lime, juiced and zested
- 1 can (14 oz) coconut milk
- 1 garlic clove, minced
- Sea salt and black pepper to taste

Instructions:
1. Heat coconut oil in a skillet over medium heat.
2. Add garlic and cook until fragrant.
3. Stir in coconut milk, lime juice, and zest. Bring to a simmer.
4. Add shrimp and cook until pink and cooked through.
5. Season with salt and pepper, and serve immediately.

Health Problems Addressed: Inflammation, nutrient deficiencies

Health Benefits: High in protein, healthy fats, and antioxidants

Scientific Benefits: Shrimp is a lean protein source; coconut milk provides healthy fats

"This shrimp dish is creamy and delicious. The coconut and lime flavors are a perfect match."

146. Balsamic Glazed Chicken

Ingredients:
- 4 chicken breasts
- 2 tablespoons olive oil
- 1/4 cup balsamic vinegar
- 2 garlic cloves, minced
- 1 tablespoon fresh rosemary, chopped
- Sea salt and black pepper to taste

Instructions:
1. Preheat the oven to 375°F (190°C).
2. In a bowl, mix olive oil, balsamic vinegar, garlic, rosemary, salt, and pepper.
3. Rub the mixture over the chicken breasts.
4. Place on a baking sheet and bake for 25-30 minutes, or until the internal temperature reaches 165°F (74°C).
5. Let rest for 5 minutes before serving.

Health Problems Addressed: Inflammation, nutrient deficiencies

Health Benefits: High in protein, antioxidants, and healthy fats

Scientific Benefits: Chicken breasts are a lean protein source; balsamic vinegar has antioxidant properties

"This chicken is tangy and flavorful. The balsamic glaze adds a nice sweetness."

147. Rosemary Garlic Lamb Chops

Ingredients:
- 4 lamb chops
- 2 tablespoons olive oil
- 4 garlic cloves, minced
- 1 tablespoon fresh rosemary, chopped
- Sea salt and black pepper to taste

Instructions:
1. In a bowl, mix olive oil, garlic, rosemary, salt, and pepper. Rub the mixture over the lamb chops.
2. Preheat grill or skillet to medium-high heat.
3. Cook lamb chops for 3-4 minutes per side for medium-rare, or until desired doneness.
4. Let rest for 5 minutes before serving.

Health Problems Addressed: Inflammation, nutrient deficiencies

Health Benefits: High in protein, healthy fats, and antioxidants

Scientific Benefits: Lamb is rich in protein and iron; rosemary has anti-inflammatory properties

"These lamb chops are juicy and delicious. The rosemary and garlic add a wonderful aroma."

148. Ginger Lime Chicken Skewers

Ingredients:
- 1 lb chicken breast, cubed
- 2 tablespoons olive oil
- 2 tablespoons fresh ginger, minced
- 1 lime, juiced and zested
- Sea salt and black pepper to taste

Instructions:
1. In a bowl, mix olive oil, ginger, lime juice, zest, salt, and pepper. Toss chicken in the mixture.
2. Thread chicken onto skewers.
3. Preheat grill to medium-high heat.
4. Grill skewers for 3-4 minutes per side, or until chicken is cooked through.
5. Serve immediately.

Health Problems Addressed: Inflammation, nutrient deficiencies

Health Benefits: High in protein, antioxidants, and vitamins

Scientific Benefits: Chicken is a lean protein source; ginger and lime have anti-inflammatory benefits

"These chicken skewers are perfect for grilling. The ginger and lime add a refreshing kick."

149. Cauliflower Rice Stir-Fry

Ingredients:
- 1 head cauliflower, grated into rice-sized pieces
- 2 tablespoons coconut oil
- 1 onion, diced
- 2 garlic cloves, minced
- 1 cup mixed vegetables (carrots, peas, bell pepper)
- 2 tablespoons coconut aminos
- Sea salt and black pepper to taste

Instructions:
1. Heat coconut oil in a large skillet over medium heat.
2. Add onion and garlic, and cook until fragrant.
3. Stir in mixed vegetables and cook until tender.

4. Add cauliflower rice, coconut aminos, salt, and pepper. Cook until the cauliflower is tender.
5. Serve immediately.

Health Problems Addressed: Inflammation, nutrient deficiencies

Health Benefits: High in vitamins, fiber, and antioxidants

Scientific Benefits: Cauliflower is low in calories and high in vitamins; mixed vegetables provide additional nutrients

"This stir-fry is a great rice alternative. The cauliflower rice is light and the vegetables are flavorful."

150. Lemon Herb Grilled Salmon

Ingredients:
- 4 salmon fillets
- 2 tablespoons olive oil
- 1 lemon, juiced and zested
- 1 tablespoon fresh dill, chopped
- 1 tablespoon fresh parsley, chopped
- Sea salt and black pepper to taste

Instructions:

1. In a bowl, mix olive oil, lemon juice, zest, dill, parsley, salt, and pepper.
2. Rub the mixture over the salmon fillets.
3. Preheat grill to medium-high heat.
4. Grill salmon for 3-4 minutes per side, or until cooked through.
5. Serve immediately.

Health Problems Addressed: Inflammation, nutrient deficiencies

Health Benefits: High in protein, omega-3 fatty acids, and antioxidants

Scientific Benefits: Salmon is rich in omega-3s; herbs have anti-inflammatory properties

"This grilled salmon is light and flavorful. The lemon and herbs add a fresh touch."

Chapter 5: Healing Snacks and Sides

151. Sweet Potato Chips

Ingredients:
- 2 large sweet potatoes, thinly sliced
- 2 tablespoons olive oil
- Sea salt to taste

Instructions:
1. Preheat the oven to 375°F (190°C).
2. Toss sweet potato slices with olive oil and sea salt.
3. Arrange slices in a single layer on a baking sheet.
4. Bake for 20-25 minutes, flipping halfway through, until crispy.
5. Let cool before serving.

Health Problems Addressed: Inflammation, nutrient deficiencies

Health Benefits: High in vitamins and antioxidants

Scientific Benefits: Sweet potatoes are rich in beta-carotene and fiber

"These sweet potato chips are a crunchy and satisfying snack."

152. Guacamole with Veggie Sticks

Ingredients:
- 3 ripe avocados
- 1 lime, juiced
- 1 small red onion, finely chopped
- 1 garlic clove, minced
- 1 small tomato, diced
- Sea salt and black pepper to taste
- Veggie sticks (carrots, celery, bell peppers) for dipping

Instructions:
1. Mash avocados in a bowl.
2. Add lime juice, red onion, garlic, tomato, salt, and pepper. Mix well.
3. Serve with veggie sticks.

Health Problems Addressed: Inflammation, nutrient deficiencies

Health Benefits: High in healthy fats, fiber, and vitamins

Scientific Benefits: Avocados are rich in monounsaturated fats and potassium

"This guacamole is creamy and flavorful. Perfect with fresh veggie sticks."

153. Coconut Yogurt with Berries

Ingredients:
- 1 cup coconut yogurt (AIP-friendly)
- 1/2 cup mixed berries (blueberries, strawberries, raspberries)
- 1 tablespoon honey (optional)

Instructions:
1. Spoon coconut yogurt into a bowl.
2. Top with mixed berries and drizzle with honey if desired.
3. Serve immediately.

Health Problems Addressed: Inflammation, gut health

Health Benefits: High in probiotics, vitamins, and antioxidants

Scientific Benefits: Coconut yogurt supports gut health; berries are rich in antioxidants

"This yogurt bowl is refreshing and healthy. A great way to start the day."

154. Zucchini Fritters

Ingredients:
- 2 large zucchinis, grated
- 1/4 cup coconut flour
- 2 eggs, beaten
- 1 garlic clove, minced
- Sea salt and black pepper to taste
- 2 tablespoons coconut oil

Instructions:
1. Squeeze excess moisture from grated zucchini.
2. In a bowl, mix zucchini, coconut flour, eggs, garlic, salt, and pepper.
3. Heat coconut oil in a skillet over medium heat.
4. Scoop zucchini mixture into the skillet and flatten into fritters.
5. Cook until golden brown, about 3-4 minutes per side.
6. Serve immediately.

Health Problems Addressed: Inflammation, nutrient deficiencies

Health Benefits: High in vitamins and fiber

Scientific Benefits: Zucchini is low in calories and high in vitamins; coconut flour is grain-free

"These fritters are crispy on the outside and tender on the inside. Delicious!"

155. Avocado Deviled Eggs

Ingredients:
- 6 hard-boiled eggs, halved
- 1 ripe avocado
- 1 tablespoon lime juice
- 1 garlic clove, minced
- Sea salt and black pepper to taste
- Paprika for garnish

Instructions:
1. Scoop out the yolks from the halved eggs.
2. In a bowl, mash yolks and avocado together.
3. Add lime juice, garlic, salt, and pepper. Mix well.
4. Spoon the mixture back into the egg whites.
5. Sprinkle it with paprika and serve.

Health Problems Addressed: Inflammation, nutrient deficiencies

Health Benefits: High in healthy fats, protein, and vitamins

Scientific Benefits: Avocados provide monounsaturated fats; eggs are a good source of protein

"These deviled eggs are creamy and flavorful. A healthier twist on a classic."

156. Kale Chips

Ingredients:
- 1 bunch kale, stems removed and leaves torn into pieces
- 2 tablespoons olive oil
- Sea salt to taste

Instructions:
1. Preheat the oven to 350°F (175°C).
2. Toss kale leaves with olive oil and sea salt.
3. Arrange leaves in a single layer on a baking sheet.
4. Bake for 10-15 minutes, or until crispy.
5. Let cool before serving.

Health Problems Addressed: Inflammation, nutrient deficiencies

Health Benefits: High in vitamins and antioxidants

Scientific Benefits: Kale is rich in vitamins A, C, and K

"These kale chips are crispy and satisfying. A great alternative to regular chips."

157. Coconut Macaroons

Ingredients:
- 2 cups unsweetened shredded coconut
- 1/2 cup coconut flour
- 1/4 cup honey
- 1/4 cup coconut oil, melted
- 1 teaspoon vanilla extract

Instructions:
1. Preheat the oven to 325°F (165°C).
2. In a bowl, mix shredded coconut, coconut flour, honey, coconut oil, and vanilla extract until well combined.
3. Scoop small amounts of the mixture and form into balls.
4. Place on a baking sheet lined with parchment paper.
5. Bake for 15-20 minutes, or until golden brown.
6. Let cool before serving.

Health Problems Addressed: Inflammation, nutrient deficiencies

Health Benefits: High in healthy fats and fiber

Scientific Benefits: Coconut products provide medium-chain triglycerides (MCTs)

"These macaroons are sweet and chewy. A perfect treat!"

158. Plantain Chips

Ingredients:
- 2 green plantains, peeled and thinly sliced
- 2 tablespoons coconut oil, melted
- Sea salt to taste

Instructions:
1. Preheat the oven to 375°F (190°C).
2. Toss plantain slices with coconut oil and sea salt.
3. Arrange slices in a single layer on a baking sheet.
4. Bake for 15-20 minutes, flipping halfway through, until crispy.
5. Let cool before serving.

Health Problems Addressed: Inflammation, nutrient deficiencies

Health Benefits: High in vitamins and antioxidants

Scientific Benefits: Plantains are rich in potassium and vitamin C

"These plantain chips are crunchy and delicious. A great snack option."

159. Carrot and Ginger Soup

Ingredients:
- 2 tablespoons coconut oil
- 1 onion, chopped
- 4 large carrots, chopped
- 1 tablespoon fresh ginger, minced
- 4 cups chicken broth (AIP-friendly)
- Sea salt and black pepper to taste

Instructions:
1. Heat coconut oil in a pot over medium heat.
2. Add onion and cook until softened.
3. Add carrots and ginger, and cook for a few minutes.
4. Pour in chicken broth and bring to a boil.
5. Reduce heat and simmer until carrots are tender.
6. Blend the soup until smooth.
7. Season with salt and pepper, and serve.

Health Problems Addressed: Inflammation, nutrient deficiencies

Health Benefits: High in vitamins and antioxidants

Scientific Benefits: Carrots are rich in beta-carotene; ginger has anti-inflammatory properties

"This soup is warm and comforting. The ginger adds a nice zing."

160. Apple Chips

Ingredients:
- 2 large apples, thinly sliced
- 1 teaspoon ground cinnamon

Instructions:
1. Preheat the oven to 225°F (110°C).
2. Arrange apple slices in a single layer on a baking sheet.
3. Sprinkle it with ground cinnamon.
4. Bake for 1.5-2 hours, or until apple slices are crispy.
5. Let cool before serving.

Health Problems Addressed: Inflammation, nutrient deficiencies

Health Benefits: High in fiber and antioxidants

Scientific Benefits: Apples are rich in fiber and vitamin C

"These apple chips are sweet and crunchy. A healthy snack option."

161. Beet Hummus

Ingredients:
- 2 medium beets, roasted and peeled
- 1 can (14 oz) chickpeas, drained and rinsed
- 2 tablespoons tahini
- 2 garlic cloves, minced
- 1 lemon, juiced
- 2 tablespoons olive oil
- Sea salt and black pepper to taste

Instructions:
1. In a food processor, blend roasted beets, chickpeas, tahini, garlic, lemon juice, olive oil, salt, and pepper until smooth.
2. Serve with veggie sticks or gluten-free crackers.

Health Problems Addressed: Inflammation, nutrient deficiencies

Health Benefits: High in fiber, vitamins, and antioxidants

Scientific Benefits: Beets are rich in nitrates; chickpeas provide plant-based protein

"This beet hummus is vibrant and delicious. A great dip for any occasion."

162. Cucumber Dill Salad

Ingredients:
- 2 large cucumbers, thinly sliced
- 1/4 cup fresh dill, chopped
- 2 tablespoons olive oil
- 1 tablespoon apple cider vinegar
- Sea salt and black pepper to taste

Instructions:
1. In a bowl, mix cucumber slices and dill.
2. In a small bowl, whisk together olive oil, apple cider vinegar, salt, and pepper.
3. Pour dressing over cucumbers and toss to coat.
4. Serve immediately or chill before serving.

Health Problems Addressed: Inflammation, nutrient deficiencies

Health Benefits: High in vitamins and antioxidants

Scientific Benefits: Cucumbers are hydrating and low in calories; dill has anti-inflammatory properties

"This cucumber salad is refreshing and light. Perfect for a summer side dish."

163. Broccoli Tots

Ingredients:
- 2 cups broccoli florets, steamed and finely chopped
- 1/4 cup coconut flour
- 1 egg, beaten
- 2 garlic cloves, minced
- Sea salt and black pepper to taste
- 2 tablespoons olive oil

Instructions:
1. Preheat the oven to 375°F (190°C).
2. In a bowl, mix chopped broccoli, coconut flour, egg, garlic, salt, and pepper.
3. Form the mixture into small tots.
4. Place on a baking sheet and drizzle with olive oil.
5. Bake for 20-25 minutes, or until golden brown.
6. Serve immediately.

Health Problems Addressed: Inflammation, nutrient deficiencies

Health Benefits: High in vitamins and fiber

Scientific Benefits: Broccoli is rich in vitamins C and K; coconut flour is grain-free

"These broccoli tots are crispy and tasty. A fun way to eat more vegetables."

164. Cauliflower Mash

Ingredients:
- 1 head cauliflower, cut into florets
- 2 tablespoons olive oil
- 1 garlic clove, minced
- Sea salt and black pepper to taste

Instructions:
1. Steam cauliflower florets until tender.
2. In a blender or food processor, blend cauliflower, olive oil, garlic, salt, and pepper until smooth.
3. Serve as a side dish.

Health Problems Addressed: Inflammation, nutrient deficiencies

Health Benefits: High in vitamins and fiber

Scientific Benefits: Cauliflower is low in calories and rich in vitamins

"This cauliflower mash is creamy and delicious. A great alternative to mashed potatoes."

165. Baked Parsnip Fries

Ingredients:
- 4 parsnips, peeled and cut into fries
- 2 tablespoons olive oil
- Sea salt and black pepper to taste

Instructions:
1. Preheat the oven to 400°F (200°C).
2. Toss parsnip fries with olive oil, salt, and pepper.
3. Arrange fries in a single layer on a baking sheet.
4. Bake for 20-25 minutes, or until golden brown.
5. Serve immediately.

Health Problems Addressed: Inflammation, nutrient deficiencies

Health Benefits: High in fiber and vitamins

Scientific Benefits: Parsnips are rich in fiber and vitamins C and K

"These parsnip fries are crispy and flavorful. A healthy alternative to regular fries."

166. Spinach Artichoke Dip

Ingredients:
- 2 cups fresh spinach, chopped
- 1 can (14 oz) artichoke hearts, drained and chopped

- 1 cup coconut cream
- 2 garlic cloves, minced
- Sea salt and black pepper to taste

Instructions:
1. Preheat the oven to 350°F (175°C).
2. In a bowl, mix spinach, artichokes, coconut cream, garlic, salt, and pepper.
3. Pour the mixture into a baking dish.
4. Bake for 20-25 minutes, or until hot and bubbly.
5. Serve with veggie sticks or gluten-free crackers.

Health Problems Addressed: Inflammation, nutrient deficiencies

Health Benefits: High in fiber, vitamins, and healthy fats

Scientific Benefits: Spinach is rich in vitamins A and K; artichokes provide antioxidants

"This dip is creamy and satisfying. Perfect for parties or gatherings."

167. Coconut Banana Bites

Ingredients:
- 2 ripe bananas, sliced
- 1/2 cup unsweetened shredded coconut

- 1 tablespoon honey (optional)

Instructions:
1. Dip banana slices in honey, if using.
2. Roll banana slices in shredded coconut.
3. Arrange on a baking sheet and freeze for 1 hour.
4. Serve immediately.

Health Problems Addressed: Inflammation, nutrient deficiencies

Health Benefits: High in vitamins and healthy fats

Scientific Benefits: Bananas are rich in potassium; coconut provides healthy fats

"These banana bites are sweet and refreshing. A perfect frozen treat."

168. Roasted Brussels Sprouts

Ingredients:
- 2 cups Brussels sprouts, halved
- 2 tablespoons olive oil
- Sea salt and black pepper to taste

Instructions:
1. Preheat the oven to 400°F (200°C).

2. Toss Brussels sprouts with olive oil, salt, and pepper.
3. Arrange in a single layer on a baking sheet.
4. Roast for 20-25 minutes, or until golden brown and tender.
5. Serve immediately.

Health Problems Addressed: Inflammation, nutrient deficiencies

Health Benefits: High in fiber, vitamins, and antioxidants

Scientific Benefits: Brussels sprouts are rich in vitamins C and K

"These roasted Brussels sprouts are crispy and delicious. A great side dish."

169. Almond Butter Stuffed Dates

Ingredients:
- 10 Medjool dates, pitted
- 1/4 cup almond butter
- Sea salt for sprinkling

Instructions:
1. Stuff each date with almond butter.
2. Sprinkle it with sea salt.
3. Serve immediately.

Health Problems Addressed: Inflammation, nutrient deficiencies

Health Benefits: High in healthy fats, fiber, and vitamins

Scientific Benefits: Dates are rich in fiber; almond butter provides healthy fats and protein

"These stuffed dates are sweet and satisfying. A great quick snack."

170. Carrot Fries

Ingredients:
- 4 large carrots, peeled and cut into fries
- 2 tablespoons olive oil
- Sea salt and black pepper to taste

Instructions:
1. Preheat the oven to 400°F (200°C).
2. Toss carrot fries with olive oil, salt, and pepper.
3. Arrange fries in a single layer on a baking sheet.
4. Bake for 20-25 minutes, or until golden brown.
5. Serve immediately.

Health Problems Addressed: Inflammation, nutrient deficiencies

Health Benefits: High in fiber and vitamins

Scientific Benefits: Carrots are rich in beta-carotene and fiber

"These carrot fries are sweet and crispy. A healthy alternative to regular fries."

171. Garlic Roasted Asparagus

Ingredients:
- 1 bunch asparagus, trimmed
- 2 tablespoons olive oil
- 2 garlic cloves, minced
- Sea salt and black pepper to taste

Instructions:
1. Preheat the oven to 400°F (200°C).
2. Toss asparagus with olive oil, garlic, salt, and pepper.
3. Arrange in a single layer on a baking sheet.
4. Roast for 15-20 minutes, or until tender.
5. Serve immediately.

Health Problems Addressed: Inflammation, nutrient deficiencies

Health Benefits: High in vitamins and antioxidants

Scientific Benefits: Asparagus is rich in vitamins A, C, and K

"This roasted asparagus is tender and flavorful. A perfect side dish."

172. Spaghetti Squash Boats

Ingredients:
- 1 large spaghetti squash, halved and seeded
- 2 tablespoons olive oil
- 1 cup marinara sauce (AIP-friendly)
- Sea salt and black pepper to taste

Instructions:
1. Preheat the oven to 400°F (200°C).
2. Drizzle spaghetti squash halves with olive oil, salt, and pepper.
3. Place cut side down on a baking sheet and bake for 30-40 minutes, or until tender.
4. Use a fork to scrape out the strands of squash.
5. Top with marinara sauce and serve.

Health Problems Addressed: Inflammation, nutrient deficiencies

Health Benefits: High in vitamins and fiber

Scientific Benefits: Spaghetti squash is low in calories and high in vitamins

"These spaghetti squash boats are a fun and healthy meal. The squash is tender and flavorful."

173. Chicken Lettuce Wraps

Ingredients:
- 1 lb ground chicken
- 2 tablespoons olive oil
- 1 onion, diced
- 2 garlic cloves, minced
- 1/4 cup coconut aminos
- 1 head butter lettuce, leaves separated
- Sea salt and black pepper to taste

Instructions:
1. Heat olive oil in a skillet over medium heat.
2. Add onion and garlic, and cook until softened.
3. Add ground chicken and cook until browned.
4. Stir in coconut aminos, salt, and pepper.
5. Spoon chicken mixture into lettuce leaves and serve.

Health Problems Addressed: Inflammation, nutrient deficiencies

Health Benefits: High in protein, vitamins, and antioxidants

Scientific Benefits: Chicken provides lean protein; lettuce is low in calories and high in vitamins

"These lettuce wraps are light and flavorful. Perfect for a quick lunch or dinner."

174. Roasted Butternut Squash

Ingredients:
- 1 large butternut squash, peeled and cubed
- 2 tablespoons olive oil
- 1 teaspoon ground cinnamon
- Sea salt to taste

Instructions:
1. Preheat the oven to 400°F (200°C).
2. Toss butternut squash cubes with olive oil, cinnamon, and sea salt.
3. Arrange in a single layer on a baking sheet.
4. Roast for 25-30 minutes, or until tender.
5. Serve immediately.

Health Problems Addressed: Inflammation, nutrient deficiencies

Health Benefits: High in vitamins and antioxidants

Scientific Benefits: Butternut squash is rich in vitamins A and C

"This roasted butternut squash is sweet and tender. A delicious side dish."

175. Cauliflower Tabbouleh

Ingredients:
- 1 head cauliflower, grated
- 1 cup cherry tomatoes, halved
- 1 cucumber, diced
- 1/4 cup fresh parsley, chopped
- 2 tablespoons olive oil
- 1 lemon, juiced
- Sea salt and black pepper to taste

Instructions:
1. In a large bowl, combine grated cauliflower, cherry tomatoes, cucumber, and parsley.
2. In a small bowl, whisk together olive oil, lemon juice, salt, and pepper.
3. Pour dressing over cauliflower mixture and toss to coat.
4. Serve immediately or chill before serving.

Health Problems Addressed: Inflammation, nutrient deficiencies

Health Benefits: High in vitamins and antioxidants

Scientific Benefits: Cauliflower is low in calories and high in vitamins; tomatoes provide antioxidants

"This tabbouleh is fresh and flavorful. A great alternative to traditional tabbouleh."

176. Apple and Walnut Salad

Ingredients:
- 4 cups mixed greens
- 1 apple, thinly sliced
- 1/2 cup walnuts, chopped
- 1/4 cup raisins
- 2 tablespoons olive oil
- 1 tablespoon apple cider vinegar
- Sea salt and black pepper to taste

Instructions:
1. In a large bowl, combine mixed greens, apple slices, walnuts, and raisins.
2. In a small bowl, whisk together olive oil, apple cider vinegar, salt, and pepper.
3. Pour dressing over salad and toss to coat.

4. Serve immediately.

Health Problems Addressed: Inflammation, nutrient deficiencies

Health Benefits: High in vitamins, healthy fats, and antioxidants

Scientific Benefits: Apples are rich in fiber and vitamin C; walnuts provide healthy fats

"This salad is crunchy and satisfying. A perfect light meal or side dish."

177. Baked Apple Slices

Ingredients:
- 4 large apples, cored and sliced
- 1 tablespoon cinnamon
- 1 tablespoon honey (optional)

Instructions:
1. Preheat the oven to 350°F (175°C).
2. Arrange apple slices in a single layer on a baking sheet.
3. Sprinkle with cinnamon and drizzle with honey if using.
4. Bake for 20-25 minutes, or until tender.

5. Serve immediately.

Health Problems Addressed: Inflammation, nutrient deficiencies

Health Benefits: High in fiber and antioxidants

Scientific Benefits: Apples are rich in fiber and vitamin C

"These baked apple slices are sweet and delicious. A great healthy dessert."

178. Roasted Carrot and Parsnip Mash

Ingredients:
- 4 large carrots, peeled and chopped
- 4 large parsnips, peeled and chopped
- 2 tablespoons olive oil
- Sea salt and black pepper to taste

Instructions:
1. Preheat the oven to 400°F (200°C).
2. Toss carrots and parsnips with olive oil, salt, and pepper.
3. Arrange in a single layer on a baking sheet.
4. Roast for 25-30 minutes, or until tender.
5. Mash roasted vegetables and serve.

Health Problems Addressed: Inflammation, nutrient deficiencies

Health Benefits: High in fiber and vitamins

Scientific Benefits: Carrots and parsnips are rich in beta-carotene and fiber

"This mash is sweet and flavorful. A great alternative to mashed potatoes."

179. Avocado and Cucumber Salad

Ingredients:
- 2 avocados, diced
- 1 large cucumber, diced
- 1/4 cup red onion, finely chopped
- 2 tablespoons olive oil
- 1 lemon, juiced
- Sea salt and black pepper to taste

Instructions:
1. In a bowl, combine diced avocados, cucumber, and red onion.
2. In a small bowl, whisk together olive oil, lemon juice, salt, and pepper.
3. Pour dressing over salad and toss to coat.

4. Serve immediately.

Health Problems Addressed: Inflammation, nutrient deficiencies

Health Benefits: High in healthy fats, vitamins, and antioxidants

Scientific Benefits: Avocados provide monounsaturated fats; cucumbers are hydrating and low in calories

"This salad is light and refreshing. Perfect for a quick and healthy snack."

180. Bacon-Wrapped Dates

Ingredients:
- 12 Medjool dates, pitted
- 12 slices of bacon

Instructions:
1. Preheat the oven to 375°F (190°C).
2. Wrap each date with a slice of bacon and secure with a toothpick.
3. Arrange on a baking sheet and bake for 15-20 minutes, or until bacon is crispy.
4. Serve immediately.

Health Problems Addressed: Inflammation, nutrient deficiencies

Health Benefits: High in healthy fats and fiber

Scientific Benefits: Dates are rich in fiber; bacon provides protein and fats

"These bacon-wrapped dates are sweet and savory. A crowd-pleasing appetizer."

181. Sweet Potato Chips

Ingredients:
- 2 large sweet potatoes, thinly sliced
- 2 tablespoons olive oil
- Sea salt to taste

Instructions:
1. Preheat the oven to 375°F (190°C).
2. Toss sweet potato slices with olive oil and sea salt.
3. Arrange in a single layer on a baking sheet.
4. Bake for 15-20 minutes, turning halfway through, until crispy.
5. Serve immediately.

Health Problems Addressed: Inflammation, nutrient deficiencies

Health Benefits: High in fiber, vitamins, and antioxidants

Scientific Benefits: Sweet potatoes are rich in beta-carotene and vitamins A and C

"These sweet potato chips are crunchy and delicious. A great alternative to store-bought chips."

182. Zucchini Fritters

Ingredients:
- 2 large zucchinis, grated
- 1 egg, beaten
- 1/4 cup coconut flour
- 2 garlic cloves, minced
- Sea salt and black pepper to taste
- 2 tablespoons olive oil

Instructions:
1. Squeeze excess moisture from grated zucchini.
2. In a bowl, mix zucchini, egg, coconut flour, garlic, salt, and pepper.
3. Heat olive oil in a skillet over medium heat.
4. Scoop batter into the skillet, forming small fritters.
5. Cook until golden brown on both sides.

6. Serve immediately.

Health Problems Addressed: Inflammation, nutrient deficiencies

Health Benefits: High in vitamins and fiber

Scientific Benefits: Zucchini is low in calories and high in vitamins

"These fritters are crispy on the outside and tender on the inside. A perfect snack."

183. Guacamole and Veggie Sticks

Ingredients:
- 2 ripe avocados, mashed
- 1 lime, juiced
- 1/4 cup red onion, finely chopped
- 1 garlic clove, minced
- Sea salt to taste
- Assorted veggie sticks (carrots, cucumbers, bell peppers)

Instructions:
1. In a bowl, mix mashed avocados, lime juice, red onion, garlic, and sea salt.
2. Serve with assorted veggie sticks.

Health Problems Addressed: Inflammation, nutrient deficiencies

Health Benefits: High in healthy fats, vitamins, and antioxidants

Scientific Benefits: Avocados provide monounsaturated fats and fiber

"This guacamole is creamy and flavorful. Perfect for dipping fresh veggies."

184. Beet Chips

Ingredients:
- 3 large beets, thinly sliced
- 2 tablespoons olive oil
- Sea salt to taste

Instructions:
1. Preheat the oven to 375°F (190°C).
2. Toss beet slices with olive oil and sea salt.
3. Arrange in a single layer on a baking sheet.
4. Bake for 20-25 minutes, turning halfway through, until crispy.
5. Serve immediately.

Health Problems Addressed: Inflammation, nutrient deficiencies

Health Benefits: High in vitamins and antioxidants

Scientific Benefits: Beets are rich in folate and antioxidants

"These beet chips are sweet and crispy. A nutritious snack."

185. Kale Chips

Ingredients:
- 1 bunch kale, stems removed and leaves torn into pieces
- 2 tablespoons olive oil
- Sea salt to taste

Instructions:
1. Preheat the oven to 350°F (175°C).
2. Toss kale pieces with olive oil and sea salt.
3. Arrange in a single layer on a baking sheet.
4. Bake for 10-15 minutes, or until crispy.
5. Serve immediately.

Health Problems Addressed: Inflammation, nutrient deficiencies

Health Benefits: High in vitamins and antioxidants

Scientific Benefits: Kale is rich in vitamins A, C, and K

"These kale chips are light and crispy. A great way to enjoy this superfood."

186. Baked Apple Chips

Ingredients:
- 4 large apples, thinly sliced
- 1 teaspoon cinnamon

Instructions:
1. Preheat the oven to 200°F (95°C).
2. Arrange apple slices in a single layer on a baking sheet.
3. Sprinkle with cinnamon.
4. Bake for 2-3 hours, or until crisp.
5. Serve immediately.

Health Problems Addressed: Inflammation, nutrient deficiencies

Health Benefits: High in fiber and antioxidants

Scientific Benefits: Apples are rich in fiber and vitamin C

"These apple chips are sweet and crunchy. A perfect healthy snack."

187. Plantain Chips

Ingredients:
- 2 green plantains, peeled and thinly sliced
- 2 tablespoons olive oil
- Sea salt to taste

Instructions:
1. Preheat the oven to 375°F (190°C).
2. Toss plantain slices with olive oil and sea salt.
3. Arrange in a single layer on a baking sheet.
4. Bake for 15-20 minutes, or until golden and crispy.
5. Serve immediately.

Health Problems Addressed: Inflammation, nutrient deficiencies

Health Benefits: High in fiber and vitamins

Scientific Benefits: Plantains are rich in vitamins A and C

"These plantain chips are crispy and delicious. A great alternative to regular chips."

188. Deviled Eggs

Ingredients:
- 6 hard-boiled eggs, peeled and halved
- 2 tablespoons olive oil
- 1 teaspoon Dijon mustard (AIP-compliant)
- Sea salt and black pepper to taste
- Paprika for garnish (optional)

Instructions:
1. Remove yolks from egg halves and place in a bowl.
2. Mash yolks with olive oil, mustard, salt, and pepper.
3. Spoon yolk mixture back into egg whites.
4. Garnish with paprika if desired.
5. Serve immediately.

Health Problems Addressed: Inflammation, nutrient deficiencies

Health Benefits: High in protein and healthy fats

Scientific Benefits: Eggs provide high-quality protein and essential vitamins

"These deviled eggs are creamy and flavorful. A perfect snack or appetizer."

189. Baked Zucchini Sticks

Ingredients:
- 2 large zucchinis, cut into sticks
- 2 tablespoons olive oil
- Sea salt and black pepper to taste

Instructions:
1. Preheat the oven to 400°F (200°C).
2. Toss zucchini sticks with olive oil, salt, and pepper.
3. Arrange in a single layer on a baking sheet.
4. Bake for 15-20 minutes, or until golden brown.
5. Serve immediately.

Health Problems Addressed: Inflammation, nutrient deficiencies

Health Benefits: High in vitamins and fiber

Scientific Benefits: Zucchini is low in calories and high in vitamins

"These zucchini sticks are crispy and tasty. A great side or snack."

190. Cabbage Rolls

Ingredients:
- 1 head cabbage, leaves separated and blanched
- 1 lb ground beef or turkey
- 1 onion, diced
- 2 garlic cloves, minced
- 1 cup cauliflower rice
- Sea salt and black pepper to taste

Instructions:
1. Preheat the oven to 350°F (175°C).
2. In a skillet, cook ground meat, onion, and garlic until browned.
3. Stir in cauliflower rice, salt, and pepper.
4. Place a spoonful of the mixture in each cabbage leaf and roll up.
5. Arrange rolls in a baking dish.
6. Bake for 25-30 minutes, or until heated through.
7. Serve immediately.

Health Problems Addressed: Inflammation, nutrient deficiencies

Health Benefits: High in protein, vitamins, and fiber

Scientific Benefits: Cabbage is rich in vitamins K and C; cauliflower rice is a low-carb alternative to grains

"These cabbage rolls are hearty and satisfying. A great meal or side dish."

191. Roasted Garlic Cauliflower

Ingredients:
- 1 head cauliflower, cut into florets
- 2 tablespoons olive oil
- 4 garlic cloves, minced
- Sea salt and black pepper to taste

Instructions:
1. Preheat the oven to 400°F (200°C).
2. Toss cauliflower florets with olive oil, garlic, salt, and pepper.
3. Arrange in a single layer on a baking sheet.
4. Roast for 20-25 minutes, or until golden and tender.
5. Serve immediately.

Health Problems Addressed: Inflammation, nutrient deficiencies

Health Benefits: High in vitamins and fiber

Scientific Benefits: Cauliflower is low in calories and high in vitamins

"This roasted garlic cauliflower is tender and flavorful. A perfect side dish."

192. Avocado Deviled Eggs

Ingredients:
- 6 hard-boiled eggs, peeled and halved
- 1 avocado, mashed
- 1 lime, juiced
- Sea salt and black pepper to taste

Instructions:
1. Remove yolks from egg halves and place in a bowl.
2. Mash yolks with avocado, lime juice, salt, and pepper.
3. Spoon avocado mixture back into egg whites.
4. Serve immediately.

Health Problems Addressed: Inflammation, nutrient deficiencies

Health Benefits: High in protein, healthy fats, and fiber

Scientific Benefits: Avocados provide monounsaturated fats and fiber; eggs offer high-quality protein

"These avocado deviled eggs are creamy and delicious. A nutritious snack."

193. Coconut Macaroons

Ingredients:
- 2 cups shredded coconut
- 2 egg whites
- 2 tablespoons honey
- 1 teaspoon vanilla extract

Instructions:
1. Preheat the oven to 350°F (175°C).
2. In a bowl, mix shredded coconut, egg whites, honey, and vanilla.
3. Scoop spoonfuls of the mixture onto a baking sheet.
4. Bake for 15-20 minutes, or until golden brown.
5. Serve immediately.

Health Problems Addressed: Inflammation, nutrient deficiencies

Health Benefits: High in healthy fats and fiber

Scientific Benefits: Coconut provides medium-chain triglycerides and fiber

"These coconut macaroons are sweet and chewy. A perfect treat."

194. Avocado Salsa

Ingredients:
- 2 avocados, diced
- 1 tomato, diced
- 1/4 cup red onion, finely chopped
- 1 lime, juiced
- Sea salt and black pepper to taste

Instructions:
1. In a bowl, combine diced avocados, tomato, and red onion.
2. Stir in lime juice, salt, and pepper.
3. Serve immediately.

Health Problems Addressed: Inflammation, nutrient deficiencies

Health Benefits: High in healthy fats, vitamins, and antioxidants

Scientific Benefits: Avocados provide monounsaturated fats and fiber

"This avocado salsa is fresh and tangy. Perfect for dipping or topping grilled meats."

195. Baked Plantain Fries

Ingredients:
- 2 ripe plantains, peeled and cut into fries
- 2 tablespoons olive oil
- Sea salt to taste

Instructions:
1. Preheat the oven to 400°F (200°C).
2. Toss plantain fries with olive oil and sea salt.
3. Arrange in a single layer on a baking sheet.
4. Bake for 20-25 minutes, turning halfway through, until golden and crispy.
5. Serve immediately.

Health Problems Addressed: Inflammation, nutrient deficiencies

Health Benefits: High in fiber and vitamins

Scientific Benefits: Plantains are rich in vitamins A and C

"These plantain fries are sweet and crispy. A great side dish or snack."

196. Cucumber and Avocado Salad

Ingredients:
- 1 large cucumber, diced

- 2 avocados, diced
- 1/4 cup fresh dill, chopped
- 1 lemon, juiced
- Sea salt and black pepper to taste

Instructions:
1. In a bowl, combine diced cucumber, avocados, and fresh dill.
2. Stir in lemon juice, salt, and pepper.
3. Serve immediately.

Health Problems Addressed: Inflammation, nutrient deficiencies

Health Benefits: High in healthy fats, vitamins, and antioxidants

Scientific Benefits: Cucumbers are hydrating and low in calories; avocados provide monounsaturated fats

"This cucumber and avocado salad is refreshing and satisfying. A perfect summer side."

197. Cauliflower Hummus

Ingredients:
- 1 head cauliflower, cut into florets
- 2 garlic cloves, minced

- 1/4 cup tahini
- 1 lemon, juiced
- Sea salt to taste
- 2 tablespoons olive oil

Instructions:
1. Steam cauliflower florets until tender.
2. In a food processor, blend steamed cauliflower, garlic, tahini, lemon juice, salt, and olive oil until smooth.
3. Serve immediately with veggie sticks.

Health Problems Addressed: Inflammation, nutrient deficiencies

Health Benefits: High in vitamins and fiber

Scientific Benefits: Cauliflower is low in calories and high in vitamins; tahini provides healthy fats

"This cauliflower hummus is creamy and delicious. A great alternative to traditional hummus."

198. Carrot and Cucumber Rolls

Ingredients:
- 2 large carrots, peeled into ribbons
- 1 large cucumber, peeled into ribbons
- 1/4 cup fresh mint leaves

- 1/4 cup fresh cilantro leaves
- 2 tablespoons olive oil
- 1 lime, juiced
- Sea salt and black pepper to taste

Instructions:
1. In a bowl, toss carrot and cucumber ribbons with mint, cilantro, olive oil, lime juice, salt, and pepper.
2. Roll up the ribbons and secure with toothpicks.
3. Serve immediately.

Health Problems Addressed: Inflammation, nutrient deficiencies

Health Benefits: High in vitamins and antioxidants

Scientific Benefits: Carrots and cucumbers are low in calories and high in vitamins

"These carrot and cucumber rolls are fresh and flavorful. A fun and healthy snack."

199. Sweet Potato and Apple Bake

Ingredients:
- 2 large sweet potatoes, peeled and sliced
- 2 large apples, peeled and sliced
- 2 tablespoons coconut oil

- 1 teaspoon cinnamon
- Sea salt to taste

Instructions:
1. Preheat the oven to 375°F (190°C).
2. In a baking dish, layer sweet potato and apple slices.
3. Drizzle with coconut oil and sprinkle with cinnamon and sea salt.
4. Bake for 30-35 minutes, or until tender.
5. Serve immediately.

Health Problems Addressed: Inflammation, nutrient deficiencies

Health Benefits: High in fiber, vitamins, and antioxidants

Scientific Benefits: Sweet potatoes are rich in beta-carotene; apples provide fiber and vitamin C

"This sweet potato and apple bake is sweet and comforting. A great side dish or dessert."

200. Garlic Roasted Mushrooms

Ingredients:
- 2 cups button mushrooms, cleaned and halved
- 2 tablespoons olive oil
- 3 garlic cloves, minced

- Sea salt and black pepper to taste

Instructions:
1. Preheat the oven to 400°F (200°C).
2. Toss mushrooms with olive oil, garlic, salt, and pepper.
3. Arrange in a single layer on a baking sheet.
4. Roast for 15-20 minutes, or until tender.
5. Serve immediately.

Health Problems Addressed: Inflammation, nutrient deficiencies

Health Benefits: High in vitamins and antioxidants

Scientific Benefits: Mushrooms are low in calories and provide essential nutrients

"These garlic roasted mushrooms are savory and delicious. A perfect side dish."

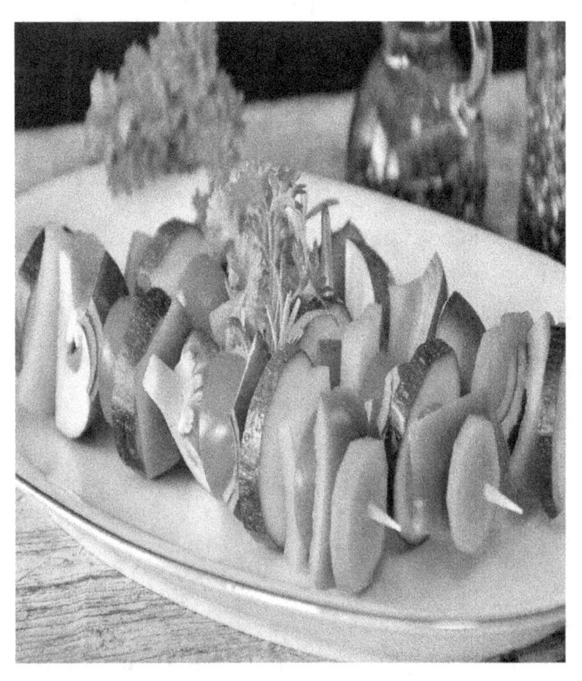

Chapter 6: Decadent Desserts

201. Chocolate Avocado Mousse

Ingredients:
- 2 ripe avocados
- 1/4 cup cocoa powder (unsweetened)
- 1/4 cup honey or maple syrup
- 1 teaspoon vanilla extract
- A pinch of sea salt

Instructions:
1. In a food processor, blend avocados until smooth.
2. Add cocoa powder, honey or maple syrup, vanilla extract, and sea salt.
3. Blend until well combined and creamy.
4. Chill for at least 30 minutes before serving.

Health Problems Addressed: Inflammation, nutrient deficiencies

Health Benefits: High in healthy fats and antioxidants

Scientific Benefits: Avocados provide monounsaturated fats and cocoa offers antioxidants

"This mousse is rich, creamy, and satisfies chocolate cravings without guilt."

202. Coconut Banana Ice Cream

Ingredients:
- 3 ripe bananas, sliced and frozen
- 1/2 cup full-fat coconut milk
- 1 teaspoon vanilla extract

Instructions:
1. In a blender, combine frozen banana slices, coconut milk, and vanilla extract.
2. Blend until smooth and creamy.
3. Serve immediately or freeze for a firmer texture.

Health Problems Addressed: Inflammation, nutrient deficiencies

Health Benefits: High in potassium and healthy fats

Scientific Benefits: Bananas provide potassium and coconut milk offers healthy fats

: "This ice cream is creamy and delicious, perfect for a hot day."

203. Apple Cinnamon Crumble

Ingredients:
- 4 large apples, peeled and sliced
- 1 teaspoon cinnamon
- 1 tablespoon honey or maple syrup
- 1/2 cup almond flour
- 1/4 cup shredded coconut
- 2 tablespoons coconut oil, melted

Instructions:
1. Preheat the oven to 350°F (175°C).
2. In a baking dish, toss apple slices with cinnamon and honey or maple syrup.
3. In a bowl, mix almond flour, shredded coconut, and melted coconut oil.
4. Sprinkle the crumble mixture over the apples.
5. Bake for 25-30 minutes, or until the topping is golden and the apples are tender.
6. Serve warm.

Health Problems Addressed: Inflammation, nutrient deficiencies

Health Benefits: High in fiber and healthy fats

Scientific Benefits: Apples provide fiber and vitamins, while almond flour offers protein and healthy fats

"This crumble is sweet and comforting, a perfect dessert for any occasion."

204. Pumpkin Pie Bars

Ingredients:
- 1 cup pumpkin puree
- 1/2 cup coconut milk
- 2 tablespoons honey or maple syrup
- 1 teaspoon cinnamon
- 1/2 teaspoon ginger
- 1/4 teaspoon nutmeg
- 1/4 teaspoon cloves
- 1/2 cup almond flour
- 1/4 cup shredded coconut
- 2 tablespoons coconut oil, melted

Instructions:
1. Preheat the oven to 350°F (175°C).
2. In a bowl, mix pumpkin puree, coconut milk, honey or maple syrup, and spices.
3. In a separate bowl, combine almond flour, shredded coconut, and melted coconut oil.
4. Press the almond flour mixture into the bottom of a baking dish to form a crust.
5. Pour the pumpkin mixture over the crust.
6. Bake for 30-35 minutes, or until set.

7. Let cool before slicing into bars.

Health Problems Addressed: Inflammation, nutrient deficiencies

Health Benefits: High in vitamins and healthy fats

Scientific Benefits: Pumpkin is rich in vitamins A and C, while almond flour offers protein and healthy fats

"These bars are rich and flavorful, capturing the essence of pumpkin pie."

205. Blueberry Coconut Bars

Ingredients:
- 2 cups fresh or frozen blueberries
- 1/4 cup honey or maple syrup
- 1 tablespoon lemon juice
- 1/2 cup shredded coconut
- 1/2 cup almond flour
- 2 tablespoons coconut oil, melted

Instructions:
1. Preheat the oven to 350°F (175°C).
2. In a saucepan, combine blueberries, honey or maple syrup, and lemon juice.

3. Cook over medium heat until the blueberries are soft and the mixture is thickened.
4. In a bowl, mix shredded coconut, almond flour, and melted coconut oil.
5. Press half of the coconut mixture into the bottom of a baking dish to form a crust.
6. Spread the blueberry mixture over the crust.
7. Sprinkle the remaining coconut mixture on top.
8. Bake for 20-25 minutes, or until the top is golden.
9. Let cool before slicing into bars.

Health Problems Addressed: Inflammation, nutrient deficiencies

Health Benefits: High in antioxidants and healthy fats

Scientific Benefits: Blueberries are rich in antioxidants, and almond flour provides protein and healthy fats

"These bars are sweet and tangy, a delightful combination of flavors."

206. Lemon Coconut Energy Balls

Ingredients:
- 1 cup shredded coconut
- 1/4 cup almond flour
- 2 tablespoons honey or maple syrup

- 1 tablespoon lemon juice
- 1 teaspoon lemon zest

Instructions:
1. In a bowl, combine shredded coconut, almond flour, honey or maple syrup, lemon juice, and lemon zest.
2. Mix until well combined.
3. Roll the mixture into small balls.
4. Chill for at least 30 minutes before serving.

Health Problems Addressed: Inflammation, nutrient deficiencies

Health Benefits: High in healthy fats and vitamins

Scientific Benefits: Coconut provides medium-chain triglycerides and fiber, while lemons offer vitamin C

"These energy balls are refreshing and satisfying, perfect for a quick snack."

207. Chocolate Coconut Macaroons

Ingredients:
- 2 cups shredded coconut
- 1/4 cup cocoa powder (unsweetened)
- 1/4 cup honey or maple syrup

- 2 egg whites
- 1 teaspoon vanilla extract

Instructions:
1. Preheat the oven to 350°F (175°C).
2. In a bowl, mix shredded coconut, cocoa powder, honey or maple syrup, egg whites, and vanilla extract.
3. Scoop spoonfuls of the mixture onto a baking sheet.
4. Bake for 15-20 minutes, or until the macaroons are set.
5. Let cool before serving.

Health Problems Addressed: Inflammation, nutrient deficiencies

Health Benefits: High in healthy fats and antioxidants

Scientific Benefits: Coconut provides medium-chain triglycerides and fiber, while cocoa offers antioxidants

"These macaroons are rich and chocolatey, a perfect indulgence."

208. Strawberry Coconut Parfaits

Ingredients:
- 2 cups fresh strawberries, sliced
- 1 cup full-fat coconut milk

- 1 tablespoon honey or maple syrup
- 1 teaspoon vanilla extract
- 1/2 cup shredded coconut

Instructions:
1. In a bowl, mix coconut milk, honey or maple syrup, and vanilla extract.
2. In serving glasses, layer strawberries, coconut milk mixture, and shredded coconut.
3. Repeat the layers until the glasses are filled.
4. Serve immediately.

Health Problems Addressed: Inflammation, nutrient deficiencies

Health Benefits: High in vitamins and healthy fats

Scientific Benefits: Strawberries provide vitamin C and antioxidants, while coconut milk offers healthy fats

"These parfaits are light and refreshing, perfect for a summer dessert."

209. Mango Coconut Pudding

Ingredients:
- 2 ripe mangoes, peeled and diced
- 1 cup full-fat coconut milk

- 2 tablespoons honey or maple syrup
- 1 teaspoon vanilla extract

Instructions:
1. In a blender, combine mangoes, coconut milk, honey or maple syrup, and vanilla extract.
2. Blend until smooth.
3. Chill for at least 1 hour before serving.

Health Problems Addressed: Inflammation, nutrient deficiencies

Health Benefits: High in vitamins and healthy fats

Scientific Benefits: Mangoes provide vitamins A and C, while coconut milk offers healthy fats

"This pudding is creamy and tropical, a delicious and healthy treat."

210. Raspberry Coconut Tarts

Ingredients:
- 1 cup fresh or frozen raspberries
- 1/4 cup honey or maple syrup
- 1 cup shredded coconut
- 1/2 cup almond flour
- 2 tablespoons coconut oil, melted

Instructions:

1. Preheat the oven to 350°F (175°C).

2. In a saucepan, combine raspberries and honey or maple syrup.

3. Cook over medium heat until the raspberries are soft and the mixture is thickened.

4. In a bowl, mix shredded coconut, almond flour, and melted coconut oil.

5. Press the coconut mixture into the bottom of tart molds to form a crust.

6. Fill the crusts with the raspberry mixture.

7. Bake for 10-15 minutes, or until the crust is golden.

8. Let cool before serving.

Health Problems Addressed: Inflammation, nutrient deficiencies

Health Benefits: High in antioxidants and healthy fats

Scientific Benefits: Raspberries provide antioxidants and fiber, while almond flour offers protein and healthy fats

"These tarts are sweet and tangy, a delightful and healthy dessert."

211. Pineapple Coconut Bars

Ingredients:
- 2 cups fresh pineapple, diced
- 1/4 cup honey or maple syrup
- 1/2 cup shredded coconut
- 1/2 cup almond flour
- 2 tablespoons coconut oil, melted

Instructions:
1. Preheat the oven to 350°F (175°C).
2. In a saucepan, combine pineapple and honey or maple syrup.
3. Cook over medium heat until the pineapple is soft and the mixture is thickened.
4. In a bowl, mix shredded coconut, almond flour, and melted coconut oil.
5. Press half of the coconut mixture into the bottom of a baking dish to form a crust.
6. Spread the pineapple mixture over the crust.
7. Sprinkle the remaining coconut mixture on top.
8. Bake for 20-25 minutes, or until the top is golden.
9. Let cool before slicing into bars.

Health Problems Addressed: Inflammation, nutrient deficiencies

Health Benefits: High in vitamins and healthy fats

Scientific Benefits: Pineapple provides vitamins C and manganese, while almond flour offers protein and healthy fats

"These bars are sweet and tropical, a refreshing and healthy treat."

212. Almond Butter Chocolate Cups

Ingredients:
- 1/2 cup almond butter
- 1/4 cup coconut oil, melted
- 1/4 cup cocoa powder (unsweetened)
- 2 tablespoons honey or maple syrup

Instructions:
1. In a bowl, mix almond butter and 1 tablespoon of melted coconut oil.
2. In a separate bowl, combine remaining coconut oil, cocoa powder, and honey or maple syrup.
3. Pour a small amount of the chocolate mixture into silicone molds to form a base.
4. Freeze for 10 minutes.
5. Add a layer of almond butter mixture on top of the chocolate base.
6. Freeze for another 10 minutes.
7. Pour the remaining chocolate mixture on top of the almond butter layer.

8. Freeze until set.

Health Problems Addressed: Inflammation, nutrient deficiencies

Health Benefits: High in healthy fats and antioxidants

Scientific Benefits: Almond butter provides protein and healthy fats, while cocoa offers antioxidants

"These chocolate cups are rich and satisfying, a perfect indulgence."

213. Banana Coconut Cookies

Ingredients:
- 2 ripe bananas, mashed
- 1 cup shredded coconut
- 1/4 cup almond flour
- 1 teaspoon vanilla extract

Instructions:
1. Preheat the oven to 350°F (175°C).
2. In a bowl, mix mashed bananas, shredded coconut, almond flour, and vanilla extract.
3. Scoop spoonfuls of the mixture onto a baking sheet.
4. Bake for 15-20 minutes, or until golden.
5. Let cool before serving.

Health Problems Addressed: Inflammation, nutrient deficiencies

Health Benefits: High in healthy fats and vitamins

Scientific Benefits: Bananas provide potassium and vitamins, while coconut offers medium-chain triglycerides and fiber

"These cookies are sweet and chewy, a delicious and healthy treat."

214. Peach Coconut Crisp

Ingredients:
- 4 large peaches, peeled and sliced
- 1/4 cup honey or maple syrup
- 1/2 cup shredded coconut
- 1/2 cup almond flour
- 2 tablespoons coconut oil, melted

Instructions:
1. Preheat the oven to 350°F (175°C).
2. In a baking dish, toss peach slices with honey or maple syrup.
3. In a bowl, mix shredded coconut, almond flour, and melted coconut oil.

4. Sprinkle the coconut mixture over the peaches.
5. Bake for 25-30 minutes, or until the topping is golden and the peaches are tender.
6. Serve warm.

Health Problems Addressed: Inflammation, nutrient deficiencies

Health Benefits: High in vitamins and healthy fats

Scientific Benefits: Peaches provide vitamins A and C, while almond flour offers protein and healthy fats

"This crisp is sweet and comforting, perfect for a summer dessert."

215. Blackberry Coconut Smoothie

Ingredients:
- 1 cup fresh or frozen blackberries
- 1 cup full-fat coconut milk
- 1 tablespoon honey or maple syrup
- 1 teaspoon vanilla extract

Instructions:
1. In a blender, combine blackberries, coconut milk, honey or maple syrup, and vanilla extract.
2. Blend until smooth.

3. Serve immediately.

Health Problems Addressed: Inflammation, nutrient deficiencies

Health Benefits: High in antioxidants and healthy fats

Scientific Benefits: Blackberries provide antioxidants and fiber, while coconut milk offers healthy fats

"This smoothie is creamy and refreshing, a perfect and healthy treat."

216. Caramelized Pineapple with Coconut Cream

Ingredients:
- 1 ripe pineapple, peeled, cored, and sliced
- 2 tablespoons coconut oil
- 2 tablespoons honey or maple syrup
- 1 cup full-fat coconut milk

Instructions:
1. In a skillet, heat coconut oil over medium heat.
2. Add pineapple slices and cook until caramelized, about 5-7 minutes per side.
3. Drizzle with honey or maple syrup.
4. Serve warm with coconut milk drizzled on top.

Health Problems Addressed: Inflammation, nutrient deficiencies

Health Benefits: High in vitamins and healthy fats

Scientific Benefits: Pineapple provides vitamins C and manganese, while coconut milk offers healthy fats

"This caramelized pineapple is sweet and tropical, a delicious and healthy dessert."

217. Fig and Walnut Bites

Ingredients:
- 1 cup dried figs, chopped
- 1/2 cup walnuts, chopped
- 2 tablespoons honey or maple syrup
- 1 teaspoon vanilla extract

Instructions:
1. In a bowl, combine chopped figs, walnuts, honey or maple syrup, and vanilla extract.
2. Roll the mixture into small balls.
3. Chill for at least 30 minutes before serving.

Health Problems Addressed: Inflammation, nutrient deficiencies

Health Benefits: High in healthy fats and fiber

Scientific Benefits: Figs provide fiber and antioxidants, while walnuts offer omega-3 fatty acids

"These bites are sweet and nutty, a perfect and healthy snack."

218. Apricot Almond Bars

Ingredients:
- 1 cup dried apricots, chopped
- 1/2 cup almond flour
- 1/4 cup shredded coconut
- 2 tablespoons coconut oil, melted
- 1 tablespoon honey or maple syrup

Instructions:
1. Preheat the oven to 350°F (175°C).
2. In a bowl, combine chopped apricots, almond flour, shredded coconut, melted coconut oil, and honey or maple syrup.
3. Press the mixture into a baking dish.
4. Bake for 20-25 minutes, or until golden.
5. Let cool before slicing into bars.

Health Problems Addressed: Inflammation, nutrient deficiencies

Health Benefits: High in vitamins and healthy fats

Scientific Benefits: Apricots provide vitamins A and C, while almond flour offers protein and healthy fats

"These bars are sweet and chewy, a delicious and healthy treat."

219. Chocolate Covered Strawberries

Ingredients:
- 1 cup fresh strawberries
- 1/2 cup dark chocolate, melted

Instructions:
1. Dip strawberries in melted dark chocolate.
2. Place on a baking sheet lined with parchment paper.
3. Chill until the chocolate is set.
4. Serve immediately.

Health Problems Addressed: Inflammation, nutrient deficiencies

Health Benefits: High in antioxidants

Scientific Benefits: Strawberries provide vitamin C and antioxidants, while dark chocolate offers antioxidants

"These chocolate covered strawberries are sweet and indulgent, a perfect and healthy dessert."

220. Pear and Almond Tart

Ingredients:
- 2 large pears, peeled and sliced
- 1/2 cup almond flour
- 1/4 cup shredded coconut
- 2 tablespoons coconut oil, melted
- 1 tablespoon honey or maple syrup

Instructions:
1. Preheat the oven to 350°F (175°C).
2. In a baking dish, arrange pear slices.
3. In a bowl, mix almond flour, shredded coconut, melted coconut oil, and honey or maple syrup.
4. Sprinkle the almond mixture over the pears.
5. Bake for 25-30 minutes, or until the topping is golden and the pears are tender.
6. Serve warm.

Health Problems Addressed: Inflammation, nutrient deficiencies

Health Benefits: High in vitamins and healthy fats

Scientific Benefits: Pears provide fiber and vitamins, while almond flour offers protein and healthy fats

"This tart is sweet and satisfying, a perfect and healthy dessert."

221. Lemon Coconut Bars

Ingredients:
- 1/2 cup coconut flour
- 1/4 cup honey or maple syrup
- 1/4 cup coconut oil, melted
- 3 eggs
- 1/2 cup lemon juice
- 1 tablespoon lemon zest

Instructions:
1. Preheat the oven to 350°F (175°C).
2. In a bowl, mix coconut flour, honey or maple syrup, and melted coconut oil.
3. Press the mixture into the bottom of a baking dish to form a crust.
4. In another bowl, whisk eggs, lemon juice, and lemon zest.
5. Pour the lemon mixture over the crust.
6. Bake for 20-25 minutes, or until set.
7. Let cool before slicing into bars.

Health Problems Addressed: Inflammation, nutrient deficiencies

Health Benefits: High in vitamins and healthy fats

Scientific Benefits: Lemons provide vitamin C and antioxidants, while coconut flour offers fiber

"These lemon bars are tangy and refreshing, a delightful and healthy treat."

222. Raspberry Almond Cookies

Ingredients:
- 1 cup almond flour
- 1/4 cup honey or maple syrup
- 1/4 cup coconut oil, melted
- 1/2 cup fresh or frozen raspberries

Instructions:
1. Preheat the oven to 350°F (175°C).
2. In a bowl, mix almond flour, honey or maple syrup, and melted coconut oil.
3. Gently fold in raspberries.
4. Scoop spoonfuls of the mixture onto a baking sheet.
5. Bake for 15-20 minutes, or until golden.
6. Let cool before serving.

Health Problems Addressed: Inflammation, nutrient deficiencies

Health Benefits: High in healthy fats and antioxidants

Scientific Benefits: Raspberries provide antioxidants and fiber, while almond flour offers protein and healthy fats

"These cookies are sweet and nutty, a delicious and healthy treat."

223. Chocolate Hazelnut Spread

Ingredients:
- 1 cup hazelnuts
- 1/4 cup cocoa powder (unsweetened)
- 1/4 cup honey or maple syrup
- 1/2 cup coconut milk
- 1 teaspoon vanilla extract

Instructions:
1. Preheat the oven to 350°F (175°C).
2. Spread hazelnuts on a baking sheet and roast for 10-15 minutes.
3. Let cool, then rub the skins off the hazelnuts.
4. In a food processor, blend hazelnuts until smooth.
5. Add cocoa powder, honey or maple syrup, coconut milk, and vanilla extract.

6. Blend until well combined.

7. Store in an airtight container in the refrigerator.

Health Problems Addressed: Inflammation, nutrient deficiencies

Health Benefits: High in healthy fats and antioxidants

Scientific Benefits: Hazelnuts provide healthy fats and protein, while cocoa offers antioxidants

"This spread is rich and creamy, perfect for a healthy and indulgent treat."

224. Cherry Coconut Smoothie Bowl

Ingredients:
- 1 cup fresh or frozen cherries
- 1/2 cup full-fat coconut milk
- 1 tablespoon honey or maple syrup
- 1 teaspoon vanilla extract
- 1/4 cup shredded coconut

Instructions:
1. In a blender, combine cherries, coconut milk, honey or maple syrup, and vanilla extract.
2. Blend until smooth.
3. Pour into a bowl and top with shredded coconut.

4. Serve immediately.

Health Problems Addressed: Inflammation, nutrient deficiencies

Health Benefits: High in antioxidants and healthy fats

Scientific Benefits: Cherries provide antioxidants and vitamins, while coconut milk offers healthy fats

"This smoothie bowl is creamy and refreshing, a perfect and healthy treat."

225. Orange Almond Cake

Ingredients:
- 2 large oranges
- 1 cup almond flour
- 1/4 cup honey or maple syrup
- 4 eggs
- 1 teaspoon baking powder
- 1 teaspoon vanilla extract

Instructions:
1. Preheat the oven to 350°F (175°C).
2. In a pot, cover oranges with water and bring to a boil. Simmer for 1 hour.
3. Drain and let the oranges cool.

4. Blend the oranges until smooth.
5. In a bowl, mix orange puree, almond flour, honey or maple syrup, eggs, baking powder, and vanilla extract.
6. Pour the batter into a greased cake pan.
7. Bake for 45-50 minutes, or until a toothpick comes out clean.
8. Let cool before serving.

Health Problems Addressed: Inflammation, nutrient deficiencies

Health Benefits: High in vitamins and healthy fats

Scientific Benefits: Oranges provide vitamin C and antioxidants, while almond flour offers protein and healthy fats

"This cake is moist and flavorful, a delicious and healthy dessert."

226. Coconut Lime Bars

Ingredients:
- 1/2 cup coconut flour
- 1/4 cup honey or maple syrup
- 1/4 cup coconut oil, melted
- 3 eggs
- 1/2 cup lime juice

- 1 tablespoon lime zest

Instructions:
1. Preheat the oven to 350°F (175°C).
2. In a bowl, mix coconut flour, honey or maple syrup, and melted coconut oil.
3. Press the mixture into the bottom of a baking dish to form a crust.
4. In another bowl, whisk eggs, lime juice, and lime zest.
5. Pour the lime mixture over the crust.
6. Bake for 20-25 minutes, or until set.
7. Let cool before slicing into bars.

Health Problems Addressed: Inflammation, nutrient deficiencies

Health Benefits: High in vitamins and healthy fats

Scientific Benefits: Limes provide vitamin C and antioxidants, while coconut flour offers fiber

"These lime bars are tangy and refreshing, a delightful and healthy treat."

227. Pomegranate Coconut Popsicles

Ingredients:
- 1 cup pomegranate juice

- 1/2 cup full-fat coconut milk
- 2 tablespoons honey or maple syrup

Instructions:
1. In a bowl, mix pomegranate juice, coconut milk, and honey or maple syrup.
2. Pour the mixture into popsicle molds.
3. Freeze for at least 4 hours, or until set.
4. Serve immediately.

Health Problems Addressed: Inflammation, nutrient deficiencies

Health Benefits: High in antioxidants and healthy fats

Scientific Benefits: Pomegranate provides antioxidants and vitamins, while coconut milk offers healthy fats

"These popsicles are sweet and refreshing, perfect for a hot day."

228. Cranberry Almond Bites

Ingredients:
- 1 cup dried cranberries
- 1/2 cup almond flour
- 1/4 cup shredded coconut
- 2 tablespoons coconut oil, melted

- 1 tablespoon honey or maple syrup

Instructions:
1. In a bowl, combine dried cranberries, almond flour, shredded coconut, melted coconut oil, and honey or maple syrup.
2. Roll the mixture into small balls.
3. Chill for at least 30 minutes before serving.

Health Problems Addressed: Inflammation, nutrient deficiencies

Health Benefits: High in antioxidants and healthy fats

Scientific Benefits: Cranberries provide antioxidants and fiber, while almond flour offers protein and healthy fats

"These bites are sweet and tart, a perfect and healthy snack."

229. Ginger Pear Crumble

Ingredients:
- 4 large pears, peeled and sliced
- 1 teaspoon ground ginger
- 1 tablespoon honey or maple syrup
- 1/2 cup almond flour
- 1/4 cup shredded coconut

- 2 tablespoons coconut oil, melted

Instructions:
1. Preheat the oven to 350°F (175°C).
2. In a baking dish, toss pear slices with ground ginger and honey or maple syrup.
3. In a bowl, mix almond flour, shredded coconut, and melted coconut oil.
4. Sprinkle the crumble mixture over the pears.
5. Bake for 25-30 minutes, or until the topping is golden and the pears are tender.
6. Serve warm.

Health Problems Addressed: Inflammation, nutrient deficiencies

Health Benefits: High in vitamins and healthy fats

Scientific Benefits: Pears provide fiber and vitamins, while almond flour offers protein and healthy fats

"This crumble is sweet and spicy, a delicious and healthy dessert."

230. Lemon Blueberry Muffins

Ingredients:
- 1 cup almond flour

- 1/4 cup coconut flour
- 1/4 cup honey or maple syrup
- 1/4 cup coconut oil, melted
- 3 eggs
- 1/2 cup blueberries
- 1 tablespoon lemon zest
- 1 teaspoon baking powder

Instructions:
1. Preheat the oven to 350°F (175°C).
2. In a bowl, mix almond flour, coconut flour, honey or maple syrup, melted coconut oil, and eggs.
3. Gently fold in blueberries, lemon zest, and baking powder.
4. Scoop the batter into a muffin tin lined with paper liners.
5. Bake for 20-25 minutes, or until a toothpick comes out clean.
6. Let cool before serving.

Health Problems Addressed: Inflammation, nutrient deficiencies

Health Benefits: High in antioxidants and healthy fats

Scientific Benefits: Blueberries provide antioxidants and fiber, while almond flour offers protein and healthy fats

"These muffins are moist and flavorful, a perfect and healthy treat."

231. Apple Cinnamon Muffins

Ingredients:
- 1 cup almond flour
- 1/4 cup coconut flour
- 1/4 cup honey or maple syrup
- 1/4 cup coconut oil, melted
- 3 eggs
- 1 apple, peeled and diced
- 1 teaspoon cinnamon
- 1 teaspoon baking powder

Instructions:
1. Preheat the oven to 350°F (175°C).
2. In a bowl, mix almond flour, coconut flour, honey or maple syrup, melted coconut oil, and eggs.
3. Fold in diced apple, cinnamon, and baking powder.
4. Scoop the batter into a muffin tin lined with paper liners.
5. Bake for 20-25 minutes, or until a toothpick comes out clean.
6. Let cool before serving.

Health Problems Addressed: Inflammation, nutrient deficiencies

Health Benefits: High in vitamins and healthy fats

Scientific Benefits: Apples provide fiber and vitamins, while cinnamon has anti-inflammatory properties

"These muffins are moist and aromatic, perfect for a healthy snack."

232. Pumpkin Spice Cake

Ingredients:
- 1 cup pumpkin puree
- 1 cup almond flour
- 1/4 cup coconut flour
- 1/4 cup honey or maple syrup
- 1/4 cup coconut oil, melted
- 3 eggs
- 1 teaspoon cinnamon
- 1/2 teaspoon nutmeg
- 1/2 teaspoon ginger
- 1 teaspoon baking powder

Instructions:
1. Preheat the oven to 350°F (175°C).
2. In a bowl, mix pumpkin puree, almond flour, coconut flour, honey or maple syrup, melted coconut oil, and eggs.

3. Add cinnamon, nutmeg, ginger, and baking powder.
4. Pour the batter into a greased cake pan.
5. Bake for 45-50 minutes, or until a toothpick comes out clean.
6. Let cool before serving.

Health Problems Addressed: Inflammation, nutrient deficiencies

Health Benefits: High in vitamins and healthy fats

Scientific Benefits: Pumpkin provides beta-carotene and vitamins, while spices have anti-inflammatory properties

"This cake is moist and flavorful, perfect for autumn."

233. Mango Coconut Pudding

Ingredients:
- 2 ripe mangoes, peeled and diced
- 1 cup full-fat coconut milk
- 2 tablespoons honey or maple syrup
- 1 teaspoon vanilla extract

Instructions:
1. In a blender, combine mangoes, coconut milk, honey or maple syrup, and vanilla extract.
2. Blend until smooth.

3. Pour into serving dishes and chill for at least 2 hours.
4. Serve cold.

Health Problems Addressed: Inflammation, nutrient deficiencies

Health Benefits: High in vitamins and healthy fats

Scientific Benefits: Mango provides vitamins A and C, while coconut milk offers healthy fats

"This pudding is creamy and tropical, a refreshing and healthy dessert."

234. Sweet Potato Brownies

Ingredients:
- 1 cup cooked sweet potato, mashed
- 1/2 cup almond flour
- 1/4 cup cocoa powder (unsweetened)
- 1/4 cup honey or maple syrup
- 1/4 cup coconut oil, melted
- 2 eggs
- 1 teaspoon vanilla extract

Instructions:
1. Preheat the oven to 350°F (175°C).

2. In a bowl, mix mashed sweet potato, almond flour, cocoa powder, honey or maple syrup, melted coconut oil, eggs, and vanilla extract.
3. Pour the batter into a greased baking dish.
4. Bake for 20-25 minutes, or until a toothpick comes out clean.
5. Let cool before slicing.

Health Problems Addressed: Inflammation, nutrient deficiencies

Health Benefits: High in vitamins and healthy fats

Scientific Benefits: Sweet potatoes provide fiber and vitamins, while cocoa offers antioxidants

"These brownies are rich and fudgy, perfect for a healthy indulgence."

235. Strawberry Basil Sorbet

Ingredients:
- 2 cups fresh strawberries, hulled
- 1/4 cup honey or maple syrup
- 1/4 cup water
- 2 tablespoons fresh basil, chopped

Instructions:

1. In a blender, combine strawberries, honey or maple syrup, water, and basil.
2. Blend until smooth.
3. Pour the mixture into an ice cream maker and churn according to the manufacturer's instructions.
4. Serve immediately or freeze until firm.

Health Problems Addressed: Inflammation, nutrient deficiencies

Health Benefits: High in vitamins and antioxidants

Scientific Benefits: Strawberries provide vitamin C and antioxidants, while basil has anti-inflammatory properties

"This sorbet is refreshing and unique, a perfect summer treat."

236. Blueberry Chia Pudding

Ingredients:
- 1 cup full-fat coconut milk
- 1/4 cup chia seeds
- 1/2 cup fresh or frozen blueberries
- 1 tablespoon honey or maple syrup
- 1 teaspoon vanilla extract

Instructions:
1. In a bowl, mix coconut milk, chia seeds, blueberries, honey or maple syrup, and vanilla extract.
2. Stir well and let sit for 10 minutes, then stir again.
3. Refrigerate for at least 2 hours or overnight.
4. Serve chilled.

Health Problems Addressed: Inflammation, nutrient deficiencies

Health Benefits: High in omega-3 fatty acids and antioxidants

Scientific Benefits: Chia seeds provide fiber and omega-3s, while blueberries offer antioxidants

"This pudding is creamy and satisfying, perfect for a healthy breakfast or dessert."

237. Avocado Lime Cheesecake

Ingredients:
- 2 ripe avocados, peeled and pitted
- 1/2 cup full-fat coconut milk
- 1/4 cup honey or maple syrup
- 1/4 cup lime juice
- 1 tablespoon lime zest
- 1 cup almond flour

- 1/4 cup shredded coconut
- 2 tablespoons coconut oil, melted

Instructions:

1. In a food processor, blend avocados, coconut milk, honey or maple syrup, lime juice, and lime zest until smooth.
2. In a bowl, mix almond flour, shredded coconut, and melted coconut oil.
3. Press the mixture into the bottom of a springform pan to form a crust.
4. Pour the avocado mixture over the crust.
5. Refrigerate for at least 4 hours or until set.
6. Serve chilled.

Health Problems Addressed: Inflammation, nutrient deficiencies

Health Benefits: High in healthy fats and vitamins

Scientific Benefits: Avocados provide healthy fats and vitamins, while lime offers vitamin C

"This cheesecake is creamy and tangy, a unique and healthy dessert."

238. Pineapple Upside-Down Cake

Ingredients:
- 1 cup fresh pineapple, sliced
- 1/4 cup honey or maple syrup
- 1/4 cup coconut oil, melted
- 3 eggs
- 1 cup almond flour
- 1/4 cup coconut flour
- 1 teaspoon baking powder
- 1 teaspoon vanilla extract

Instructions:
1. Preheat the oven to 350°F (175°C).
2. In a baking dish, arrange pineapple slices in a single layer.
3. Drizzle honey or maple syrup over the pineapple.
4. In a bowl, mix coconut oil, eggs, almond flour, coconut flour, baking powder, and vanilla extract.
5. Pour the batter over the pineapple slices.
6. Bake for 30-35 minutes, or until a toothpick comes out clean.
7. Let cool for 10 minutes, then invert onto a serving plate.
8. Serve warm.

Health Problems Addressed: Inflammation, nutrient deficiencies

Health Benefits: High in vitamins and healthy fats

Scientific Benefits: Pineapple provides vitamins C and manganese, while almond flour offers protein and healthy fats

"This cake is sweet and fruity, perfect for a healthy dessert."

239. Carrot Cake Energy Balls

Ingredients:
- 1 cup shredded carrots
- 1/2 cup almond flour
- 1/4 cup shredded coconut
- 2 tablespoons honey or maple syrup
- 1 teaspoon cinnamon
- 1/2 teaspoon nutmeg

Instructions:
1. In a bowl, combine shredded carrots, almond flour, shredded coconut, honey or maple syrup, cinnamon, and nutmeg.
2. Roll the mixture into small balls.
3. Chill for at least 30 minutes before serving.

Health Problems Addressed: Inflammation, nutrient deficiencies

Health Benefits: High in vitamins and healthy fats

Scientific Benefits: Carrots provide beta-carotene and vitamins, while spices have anti-inflammatory properties

"These energy balls are sweet and spicy, perfect for a healthy snack."

240. Raspberry Coconut Macaroons

Ingredients:
- 2 cups shredded coconut
- 1/2 cup fresh or frozen raspberries
- 1/4 cup honey or maple syrup
- 2 egg whites
- 1 teaspoon vanilla extract

Instructions:
1. Preheat the oven to 350°F (175°C).
2. In a bowl, mix shredded coconut, raspberries, honey or maple syrup, egg whites, and vanilla extract.
3. Scoop spoonfuls of the mixture onto a baking sheet.
4. Bake for 15-20 minutes, or until golden.
5. Let cool before serving.

Health Problems Addressed: Inflammation, nutrient deficiencies

Health Benefits: High in healthy fats and antioxidants

Scientific Benefits: Raspberries provide antioxidants and fiber, while coconut offers healthy fats

"These macaroons are sweet and chewy, perfect for a healthy treat."

241. Peach Basil Cobbler

Ingredients:
- 4 large peaches, peeled and sliced
- 1/4 cup honey or maple syrup
- 2 tablespoons fresh basil, chopped
- 1 cup almond flour
- 1/4 cup shredded coconut
- 2 tablespoons coconut oil, melted

Instructions:
1. Preheat the oven to 350°F (175°C).
2. In a baking dish, toss peach slices with honey or maple syrup and basil.
3. In a bowl, mix almond flour, shredded coconut, and melted coconut oil.
4. Sprinkle the crumble mixture over the peaches.
5. Bake for 25-30 minutes, or until the topping is golden and the peaches are tender.
6. Serve warm.

Health Problems Addressed: Inflammation, nutrient deficiencies

Health Benefits: High in vitamins and healthy fats

Scientific Benefits: Peaches provide fiber and vitamins, while basil has anti-inflammatory properties

"This cobbler is sweet and fragrant, perfect for a healthy dessert."

242. Chocolate Orange Truffles

Ingredients:
- 1 cup almond flour
- 1/4 cup cocoa powder (unsweetened)
- 1/4 cup honey or maple syrup
- 1/4 cup coconut oil, melted
- 1 tablespoon orange zest

Instructions:
1. In a bowl, mix almond flour, cocoa powder, honey or maple syrup, melted coconut oil, and orange zest.
2. Roll the mixture into small balls.
3. Chill for at least 30 minutes before serving.

Health Problems Addressed: Inflammation, nutrient deficiencies

Health Benefits: High in healthy fats and antioxidants

Scientific Benefits: Cocoa provides antioxidants, while orange zest offers vitamin C

"These truffles are rich and zesty, perfect for a healthy treat."

243. Blackberry Lime Parfait

Ingredients:
- 1 cup fresh or frozen blackberries
- 1/4 cup honey or maple syrup
- 1 cup full-fat coconut yogurt
- 1 tablespoon lime zest

Instructions:
1. In a bowl, mix blackberries with honey or maple syrup.
2. In serving glasses, layer coconut yogurt and blackberry mixture.
3. Sprinkle it with lime zest.
4. Serve immediately.

Health Problems Addressed: Inflammation, nutrient deficiencies

Health Benefits: High in antioxidants and healthy fats

Scientific Benefits: Blackberries provide antioxidants and vitamins, while coconut yogurt offers healthy fats

"This parfait is creamy and tangy, perfect for a healthy dessert."

244. Plum Almond Tart

Ingredients:
- 4 large plums, sliced
- 1/4 cup honey or maple syrup
- 1 cup almond flour
- 1/4 cup shredded coconut
- 2 tablespoons coconut oil, melted
- 1 teaspoon vanilla extract

Instructions:
1. Preheat the oven to 350°F (175°C).
2. In a bowl, toss plum slices with honey or maple syrup.
3. In another bowl, mix almond flour, shredded coconut, melted coconut oil, and vanilla extract.
4. Press the mixture into the bottom of a tart pan to form a crust.

5. Arrange plum slices over the crust.

6. Bake for 25-30 minutes, or until the plums are tender.

7. Let cool before serving.

Health Problems Addressed: Inflammation, nutrient deficiencies

Health Benefits: High in vitamins and healthy fats

Scientific Benefits: Plums provide fiber and vitamins, while almond flour offers protein and healthy fats

"This tart is sweet and fruity, perfect for a healthy dessert."

245. Banana Walnut Bread

Ingredients:
- 3 ripe bananas, mashed
- 1 cup almond flour
- 1/4 cup coconut flour
- 1/4 cup honey or maple syrup
- 1/4 cup coconut oil, melted
- 3 eggs
- 1/2 cup chopped walnuts
- 1 teaspoon baking powder
- 1 teaspoon vanilla extract

Instructions:
1. Preheat the oven to 350°F (175°C).
2. In a bowl, mix mashed bananas, almond flour, coconut flour, honey or maple syrup, melted coconut oil, eggs, walnuts, baking powder, and vanilla extract.
3. Pour the batter into a greased loaf pan.
4. Bake for 45-50 minutes, or until a toothpick comes out clean.
5. Let cool before slicing.

Health Problems Addressed: Inflammation, nutrient deficiencies

Health Benefits: High in healthy fats and vitamins

Scientific Benefits: Bananas provide potassium and vitamins, while walnuts offer healthy fats and protein

"This bread is moist and nutty, perfect for a healthy snack."

246. Fig and Walnut Tart

Ingredients:
- 1 cup dried figs, chopped
- 1/2 cup walnuts, chopped
- 1/4 cup honey or maple syrup
- 1 cup almond flour

- 1/4 cup shredded coconut
- 2 tablespoons coconut oil, melted
- 1 teaspoon vanilla extract

Instructions:
1. Preheat the oven to 350°F (175°C).
2. In a bowl, mix chopped figs, walnuts, and honey or maple syrup.
3. In another bowl, mix almond flour, shredded coconut, melted coconut oil, and vanilla extract.
4. Press the mixture into the bottom of a tart pan to form a crust.
5. Spread the fig and walnut mixture over the crust.
6. Bake for 20-25 minutes, or until the tart is golden.
7. Let cool before serving.

Health Problems Addressed: Inflammation, nutrient deficiencies

Health Benefits: High in healthy fats and vitamins

Scientific Benefits: Figs provide fiber and vitamins, while walnuts offer healthy fats and protein

"This tart is sweet and nutty, perfect for a healthy dessert."

247. Lemon Thyme Shortbread

Ingredients:
- 1 cup almond flour
- 1/4 cup coconut flour
- 1/4 cup honey or maple syrup
- 1/4 cup coconut oil, melted
- 1 tablespoon lemon zest
- 1 teaspoon fresh thyme, chopped

Instructions:
1. Preheat the oven to 350°F (175°C).
2. In a bowl, mix almond flour, coconut flour, honey or maple syrup, melted coconut oil, lemon zest, and thyme.
3. Roll the dough into a log and slice into rounds.
4. Place the rounds on a baking sheet.
5. Bake for 15-20 minutes, or until golden.
6. Let cool before serving.

Health Problems Addressed: Inflammation, nutrient deficiencies

Health Benefits: High in healthy fats and antioxidants

Scientific Benefits: Lemon provides vitamin C and antioxidants, while thyme has anti-inflammatory properties

"These shortbread cookies are buttery and fragrant, perfect for a healthy treat."

248. Apricot Coconut Bars

Ingredients:
- 1 cup dried apricots, chopped
- 1/2 cup shredded coconut
- 1/4 cup honey or maple syrup
- 1/4 cup coconut oil, melted
- 1 cup almond flour
- 1 teaspoon vanilla extract

Instructions:
1. Preheat the oven to 350°F (175°C).
2. In a bowl, mix chopped apricots, shredded coconut, honey or maple syrup, melted coconut oil, almond flour, and vanilla extract.
3. Press the mixture into the bottom of a baking dish.
4. Bake for 20-25 minutes, or until golden.
5. Let cool before slicing into bars.

Health Problems Addressed: Inflammation, nutrient deficiencies

Health Benefits: High in healthy fats and vitamins

Scientific Benefits: Apricots provide fiber and vitamins, while coconut offers healthy fats

"These bars are sweet and chewy, perfect for a healthy snack."

249. Apple Pecan Crisp

Ingredients:
- 4 large apples, peeled and sliced
- 1/4 cup honey or maple syrup
- 1/2 cup pecans, chopped
- 1 cup almond flour
- 1/4 cup shredded coconut
- 2 tablespoons coconut oil, melted
- 1 teaspoon cinnamon

Instructions:
1. Preheat the oven to 350°F (175°C).
2. In a baking dish, toss apple slices with honey or maple syrup.
3. In a bowl, mix chopped pecans, almond flour, shredded coconut, melted coconut oil, and cinnamon.
4. Sprinkle the crisp mixture over the apples.
5. Bake for 25-30 minutes, or until the topping is golden and the apples are tender.
6. Serve warm.

Health Problems Addressed: Inflammation, nutrient deficiencies

Health Benefits: High in healthy fats and vitamins

Scientific Benefits: Apples provide fiber and vitamins, while pecans offer healthy fats and protein

"This crisp is sweet and nutty, perfect for a healthy dessert."

250. Kiwi Lime Popsicles

Ingredients:
- 4 ripe kiwis, peeled and sliced
- 1/4 cup honey or maple syrup
- 1/4 cup lime juice
- 1 tablespoon lime zest

Instructions:
1. In a blender, combine kiwis, honey or maple syrup, lime juice, and lime zest.
2. Blend until smooth.
3. Pour the mixture into popsicle molds.
4. Freeze for at least 4 hours or until solid.
5. Serve cold.

Health Problems Addressed: Inflammation, nutrient deficiencies

Health Benefits: High in vitamins and antioxidants

Scientific Benefits: Kiwis provide vitamin C and antioxidants, while lime offers vitamin C

"These popsicles are tangy and refreshing, perfect for a healthy treat."

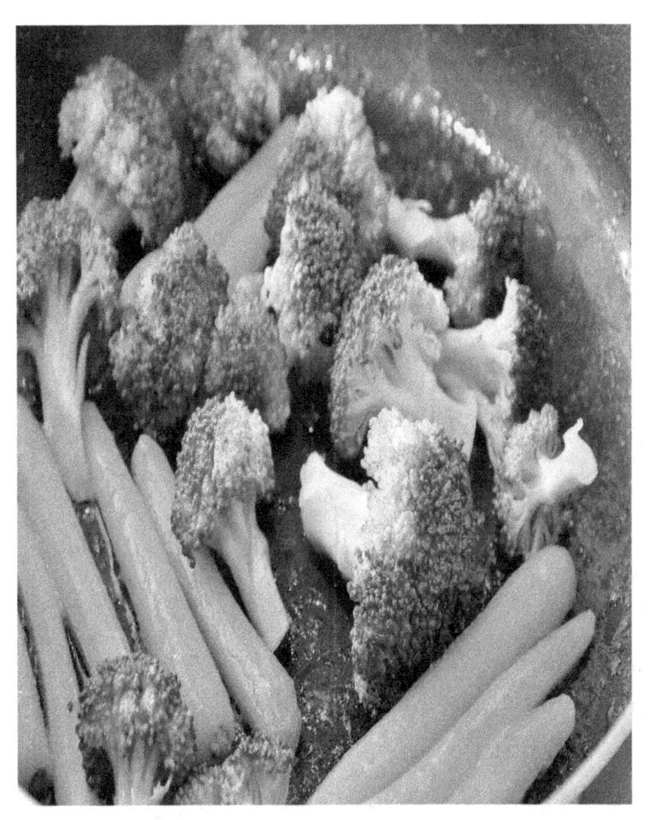

Chapter 7: Essential Sauces and Condiments

251. Tangy Lemon Herb Dressing

Ingredients:
- 1/4 cup olive oil
- 2 tablespoons fresh lemon juice
- 1 teaspoon Dijon mustard (AIP compliant)
- 1 clove garlic, minced
- 1 tablespoon fresh parsley, chopped
- Salt and pepper to taste

Instructions:
1. In a bowl, whisk together olive oil, lemon juice, Dijon mustard, and garlic.
2. Stir in chopped parsley.
3. Season with salt and pepper to taste.
4. Store in the refrigerator for up to one week.

Health Problems Addressed: Inflammation, nutrient deficiencies

Health Benefits: High in healthy fats and antioxidants

Scientific Benefits: Olive oil provides healthy fats, and lemon juice offers vitamin C and antioxidants

"This dressing is refreshing and versatile, perfect for salads and marinades."

252. Creamy Avocado Cilantro Sauce

Ingredients:
- 2 ripe avocados, peeled and pitted
- 1/4 cup fresh cilantro, chopped
- 1/4 cup lime juice
- 1/4 cup olive oil
- 1 clove garlic, minced
- Salt and pepper to taste

Instructions:
1. In a blender, combine avocados, cilantro, lime juice, olive oil, and garlic.
2. Blend until smooth.
3. Season with salt and pepper to taste.
4. Store in the refrigerator for up to three days.

Health Problems Addressed: Inflammation, nutrient deficiencies

Health Benefits: High in healthy fats and vitamins

Scientific Benefits: Avocados provide healthy fats and vitamins, while cilantro has antioxidant properties

"This sauce is creamy and flavorful, perfect for tacos and salads."

253. Sweet and Smoky Barbecue Sauce

Ingredients:
- 1 cup tomato puree
- 1/4 cup apple cider vinegar
- 1/4 cup honey or maple syrup
- 2 tablespoons coconut aminos
- 1 teaspoon smoked paprika
- 1/2 teaspoon garlic powder
- 1/2 teaspoon onion powder

Instructions:
1. In a saucepan, combine tomato puree, apple cider vinegar, honey or maple syrup, and coconut aminos.
2. Add smoked paprika, garlic powder, and onion powder.
3. Simmer over low heat for 20 minutes, stirring occasionally.
4. Store in the refrigerator for up to two weeks.

Health Problems Addressed: Inflammation

Health Benefits: Low in sugar and high in antioxidants

Scientific Benefits: Tomatoes provide lycopene and vitamins, while apple cider vinegar has anti-inflammatory properties

"This barbecue sauce is sweet, smoky, and perfect for grilling."

254. Zesty Ginger Garlic Sauce

Ingredients:
- 1/4 cup coconut aminos
- 1/4 cup apple cider vinegar
- 2 tablespoons fresh ginger, grated
- 2 cloves garlic, minced
- 1 tablespoon honey or maple syrup
- 1/4 teaspoon red pepper flakes (optional)

Instructions:
1. In a bowl, combine coconut aminos, apple cider vinegar, ginger, garlic, honey or maple syrup, and red pepper flakes (if using).
2. Mix well.
3. Store in the refrigerator for up to one week.

Health Problems Addressed: Inflammation, digestive issues

Health Benefits: High in antioxidants and anti-inflammatory compounds

Scientific Benefits: Ginger and garlic have powerful anti-inflammatory and antioxidant properties

"This sauce is spicy and zesty, perfect for stir-fries and marinades."

255. Classic Basil Pesto

Ingredients:
- 2 cups fresh basil leaves
- 1/4 cup pine nuts or walnuts
- 2 cloves garlic
- 1/2 cup olive oil
- 1/4 cup nutritional yeast
- Salt and pepper to taste

Instructions:
1. In a food processor, combine basil leaves, nuts, and garlic.
2. Pulse until finely chopped.
3. With the processor running, slowly add olive oil until the mixture is smooth.
4. Stir in nutritional yeast.
5. Season with salt and pepper to taste.

6. Store in the refrigerator for up to one week.

Health Problems Addressed: Inflammation, nutrient deficiencies

Health Benefits: High in healthy fats and antioxidants

Scientific Benefits: Basil provides antioxidants, and nuts offer healthy fats and protein

"This pesto is fresh and aromatic, perfect for pasta and sandwiches."

256. Spicy Mango Chutney

Ingredients:
- 2 ripe mangoes, peeled and diced
- 1/4 cup apple cider vinegar
- 1/4 cup honey or maple syrup
- 1 small onion, finely chopped
- 1 clove garlic, minced
- 1 teaspoon grated fresh ginger
- 1/2 teaspoon red pepper flakes

Instructions:
1. In a saucepan, combine mangoes, apple cider vinegar, honey or maple syrup, onion, garlic, ginger, and red pepper flakes.

2. Simmer over low heat for 30 minutes, stirring occasionally.
3. Store in the refrigerator for up to two weeks.

Health Problems Addressed: Inflammation

Health Benefits: High in vitamins and antioxidants

Scientific Benefits: Mangoes provide vitamins A and C, and ginger has anti-inflammatory properties

"This chutney is sweet, spicy, and perfect for adding a kick to meals."

257. Roasted Red Pepper Dip

Ingredients:
- 2 large red bell peppers, roasted and peeled
- 1/4 cup olive oil
- 2 cloves garlic, minced
- 1 tablespoon fresh lemon juice
- 1 teaspoon smoked paprika
- Salt and pepper to taste

Instructions:
1. In a blender, combine roasted red peppers, olive oil, garlic, lemon juice, and smoked paprika.
2. Blend until smooth.

3. Season with salt and pepper to taste.
4. Store in the refrigerator for up to one week.

Health Problems Addressed: Inflammation

Health Benefits: High in vitamins and antioxidants

Scientific Benefits: Red bell peppers provide vitamins C and A, and olive oil offers healthy fats

"This dip is smoky and creamy, perfect for vegetables and crackers."

258. Creamy Cashew Alfredo Sauce

Ingredients:
- 1 cup raw cashews, soaked overnight and drained
- 1/2 cup water
- 1/4 cup nutritional yeast
- 2 cloves garlic, minced
- 2 tablespoons lemon juice
- Salt and pepper to taste

Instructions:
1. In a blender, combine soaked cashews, water, nutritional yeast, garlic, and lemon juice.
2. Blend until smooth.
3. Season with salt and pepper to taste.

4. Store in the refrigerator for up to one week.

Health Problems Addressed: Inflammation, nutrient deficiencies

Health Benefits: High in healthy fats and vitamins

Scientific Benefits: Cashews provide protein and healthy fats, and nutritional yeast offers B vitamins

"This Alfredo sauce is rich and creamy, perfect for pasta and vegetables."

259. Honey Mustard Dressing

Ingredients:
- 1/4 cup Dijon mustard (AIP compliant)
- 1/4 cup honey
- 2 tablespoons apple cider vinegar
- 1/4 cup olive oil
- Salt and pepper to taste

Instructions:
1. In a bowl, whisk together Dijon mustard, honey, apple cider vinegar, and olive oil.
2. Season with salt and pepper to taste.
3. Store in the refrigerator for up to one week.

Health Problems Addressed: Inflammation

Health Benefits: High in antioxidants and healthy fats

Scientific Benefits: Mustard provides antioxidants, and olive oil offers healthy fats

"This dressing is tangy and sweet, perfect for salads and marinades."

260. Turmeric Tahini Sauce

Ingredients:
- 1/2 cup tahini
- 1/4 cup water
- 2 tablespoons lemon juice
- 1 teaspoon ground turmeric
- 1 clove garlic, minced
- Salt and pepper to taste

Instructions:
1. In a bowl, whisk together tahini, water, lemon juice, turmeric, and garlic.
2. Season with salt and pepper to taste.
3. Store in the refrigerator for up to one week.

Health Problems Addressed: Inflammation

Health Benefits: High in healthy fats and antioxidants

Scientific Benefits: Tahini provides healthy fats and protein, and turmeric has anti-inflammatory properties

"This sauce is creamy and earthy, perfect for drizzling over roasted vegetables."

261. Chimichurri Sauce

Ingredients:
- 1 cup fresh parsley, chopped
- 1/4 cup fresh cilantro, chopped
- 1/4 cup olive oil
- 2 tablespoons red wine vinegar
- 2 cloves garlic, minced
- 1 teaspoon dried oregano
- Salt and pepper to taste

Instructions:
1. In a bowl, combine parsley, cilantro, olive oil, red wine vinegar, garlic, and oregano.
2. Mix well.
3. Season with salt and pepper to taste.
4. Store in the refrigerator for up to one week.

Health Problems Addressed: Inflammation

Health Benefits: High in antioxidants and healthy fats

Scientific Benefits: Parsley and cilantro provide vitamins and antioxidants, and olive oil offers healthy fats

"This chimichurri is fresh and tangy, perfect for grilled meats and vegetables."

262. Beetroot Hummus

Ingredients:
- 2 medium beets, roasted and peeled
- 1/4 cup tahini
- 2 tablespoons lemon juice
- 2 cloves garlic, minced
- 1/4 cup olive oil
- Salt and pepper to taste

Instructions:
1. In a blender, combine roasted beets, tahini, lemon juice, garlic, and olive oil.
2. Blend until smooth.
3. Season with salt and pepper to taste.
4. Store in the refrigerator for up to one week.

Health Problems Addressed: Inflammation, nutrient deficiencies

Health Benefits: High in vitamins and antioxidants

Scientific Benefits: Beets provide antioxidants and vitamins, and tahini offers healthy fats and protein

"This hummus is vibrant and earthy, perfect for dipping vegetables and spreading on sandwiches."

263. Spicy Sriracha Mayo

Ingredients:
- 1/2 cup mayonnaise (AIP compliant)
- 2 tablespoons sriracha sauce (AIP compliant)
- 1 tablespoon lime juice

Instructions:
1. In a bowl, whisk together mayonnaise, sriracha sauce, and lime juice.
2. Store in the refrigerator for up to one week.

Health Problems Addressed: Inflammation

Health Benefits: High in healthy fats

Scientific Benefits: Sriracha provides capsaicin, which has anti-inflammatory properties

"This mayo is spicy and creamy, perfect for burgers and sandwiches."

264. Classic Vinaigrette

Ingredients:
- 1/4 cup olive oil
- 2 tablespoons apple cider vinegar
- 1 teaspoon Dijon mustard (AIP compliant)
- 1 clove garlic, minced
- Salt and pepper to taste

Instructions:
1. In a bowl, whisk together olive oil, apple cider vinegar, Dijon mustard, and garlic.
2. Season with salt and pepper to taste.
3. Store in the refrigerator for up to one week.

Health Problems Addressed: Inflammation

Health Benefits: High in healthy fats and antioxidants

Scientific Benefits: Olive oil provides healthy fats, and apple cider vinegar has anti-inflammatory properties

"This vinaigrette is classic and versatile, perfect for salads and marinades."

265. Mint Coconut Chutney

Ingredients:
- 1 cup fresh mint leaves
- 1/4 cup shredded coconut
- 2 tablespoons lime juice
- 1 clove garlic, minced
- 1 tablespoon honey or maple syrup
- Salt to taste

Instructions:
1. In a blender, combine mint leaves, shredded coconut, lime juice, garlic, and honey or maple syrup.
2. Blend until smooth.
3. Season with salt to taste.
4. Store in the refrigerator for up to one week.

Health Problems Addressed: Inflammation, digestive issues

Health Benefits: High in vitamins and antioxidants

Scientific Benefits: Mint provides antioxidants and aids digestion, and coconut offers healthy fats

"This chutney is refreshing and sweet, perfect for adding a burst of flavor to dishes."

266. Garlic Herb Aioli

Ingredients:
- 1/2 cup mayonnaise (AIP compliant)
- 2 cloves garlic, minced
- 1 tablespoon fresh lemon juice
- 1 tablespoon fresh parsley, chopped
- 1 tablespoon fresh dill, chopped
- Salt and pepper to taste

Instructions:
1. In a bowl, whisk together mayonnaise, garlic, lemon juice, parsley, and dill.
2. Season with salt and pepper to taste.
3. Store in the refrigerator for up to one week.

Health Problems Addressed: Inflammation

Health Benefits: High in healthy fats

Scientific Benefits: Garlic has anti-inflammatory and antimicrobial properties

"This aioli is creamy and herby, perfect for dipping vegetables or spreading on sandwiches."

267. Pineapple Salsa

Ingredients:
- 1 cup fresh pineapple, diced
- 1/4 cup red onion, finely chopped
- 1/4 cup fresh cilantro, chopped
- 1 jalapeño, seeded and finely chopped
- 2 tablespoons lime juice
- Salt to taste

Instructions:
1. In a bowl, combine pineapple, red onion, cilantro, jalapeño, and lime juice.
2. Mix well.
3. Season with salt to taste.
4. Store in the refrigerator for up to three days.

Health Problems Addressed: Inflammation

Health Benefits: High in vitamins and antioxidants

Scientific Benefits: Pineapple contains bromelain, which has anti-inflammatory properties

"This salsa is sweet, tangy, and perfect for topping grilled meats or fish."

268. Roasted Garlic and Beet Dip

Ingredients:

- 2 medium beets, roasted and peeled
- 1 head of garlic, roasted
- 1/4 cup tahini
- 2 tablespoons lemon juice
- 1/4 cup olive oil
- Salt and pepper to taste

Instructions:

1. In a blender, combine roasted beets, roasted garlic, tahini, lemon juice, and olive oil.
2. Blend until smooth.
3. Season with salt and pepper to taste.
4. Store in the refrigerator for up to one week.

Health Problems Addressed: Inflammation, nutrient deficiencies

Health Benefits: High in vitamins and antioxidants

Scientific Benefits: Beets provide antioxidants and vitamins, and garlic has anti-inflammatory properties

"This dip is earthy and creamy, perfect for vegetables and crackers."

269. Coconut Curry Sauce

Ingredients:

- 1 can full-fat coconut milk
- 1 tablespoon curry powder
- 1 tablespoon fresh ginger, grated
- 2 cloves garlic, minced
- 1 tablespoon lime juice
- Salt and pepper to taste

Instructions:
1. In a saucepan, combine coconut milk, curry powder, ginger, garlic, and lime juice.
2. Simmer over low heat for 10 minutes, stirring occasionally.
3. Season with salt and pepper to taste.
4. Store in the refrigerator for up to one week.

Health Problems Addressed: Inflammation, digestive issues

Health Benefits: High in healthy fats and anti-inflammatory compounds

Scientific Benefits: Coconut milk provides healthy fats, and curry powder has anti-inflammatory properties

"This curry sauce is rich and flavorful, perfect for vegetables and meats."

270. Sesame Ginger Dressing

Ingredients:
- 1/4 cup olive oil
- 2 tablespoons coconut aminos
- 1 tablespoon fresh ginger, grated
- 1 clove garlic, minced
- 1 tablespoon sesame oil
- 1 tablespoon lime juice
- Salt and pepper to taste

Instructions:
1. In a bowl, whisk together olive oil, coconut aminos, ginger, garlic, sesame oil, and lime juice.
2. Season with salt and pepper to taste.
3. Store in the refrigerator for up to one week.

Health Problems Addressed: Inflammation, digestive issues

Health Benefits: High in healthy fats and antioxidants

Scientific Benefits: Ginger and garlic have anti-inflammatory and digestive properties

"This dressing is zesty and nutty, perfect for salads and marinades."

271. Spicy Harissa Sauce

Ingredients:
- 2 roasted red bell peppers, peeled and seeded
- 2 tablespoons olive oil
- 1 tablespoon apple cider vinegar
- 1 teaspoon smoked paprika
- 1 teaspoon ground cumin
- 1/2 teaspoon cayenne pepper
- 2 cloves garlic, minced
- Salt to taste

Instructions:
1. In a blender, combine roasted red bell peppers, olive oil, apple cider vinegar, smoked paprika, cumin, cayenne pepper, and garlic.
2. Blend until smooth.
3. Season with salt to taste.
4. Store in the refrigerator for up to one week.

Health Problems Addressed: Inflammation

Health Benefits: High in antioxidants and anti-inflammatory compounds

Scientific Benefits: Bell peppers provide vitamins and antioxidants, and spices like cumin and paprika have anti-inflammatory properties

"This harissa is spicy and flavorful, perfect for adding heat to dishes."

272. Fresh Cucumber Dill Sauce

Ingredients:
- 1 cup cucumber, grated and drained
- 1/2 cup coconut yogurt (AIP compliant)
- 1 tablespoon fresh dill, chopped
- 1 tablespoon lemon juice
- 1 clove garlic, minced
- Salt and pepper to taste

Instructions:
1. In a bowl, combine grated cucumber, coconut yogurt, dill, lemon juice, and garlic.
2. Mix well.
3. Season with salt and pepper to taste.
4. Store in the refrigerator for up to three days.

Health Problems Addressed: Inflammation, digestive issues

Health Benefits: Cooling and hydrating

Scientific Benefits: Cucumbers are hydrating and soothing for the digestive system

"This sauce is refreshing and creamy, perfect for dipping vegetables or as a topping for meats."

273. Zesty Orange Ginger Glaze

Ingredients:
- 1/2 cup orange juice
- 1 tablespoon fresh ginger, grated
- 1 tablespoon honey or maple syrup
- 1 tablespoon coconut aminos
- 1 teaspoon arrowroot powder

Instructions:
1. In a saucepan, combine orange juice, ginger, honey or maple syrup, and coconut aminos.
2. Bring to a simmer over medium heat.
3. In a small bowl, dissolve arrowroot powder in a little water and add to the saucepan.
4. Stir until the glaze thickens.
5. Store in the refrigerator for up to one week.

Health Problems Addressed: Inflammation

Health Benefits: High in vitamins and antioxidants

Scientific Benefits: Orange juice provides vitamin C, and ginger has anti-inflammatory properties

"This glaze is tangy and sweet, perfect for glazing meats or vegetables."

274. Savory Mushroom Gravy

Ingredients:
- 2 cups mushrooms, sliced
- 1/4 cup onion, finely chopped
- 2 cloves garlic, minced
- 1 tablespoon olive oil
- 2 cups bone broth
- 1 tablespoon arrowroot powder
- 1 tablespoon coconut aminos
- Salt and pepper to taste

Instructions:
1. In a saucepan, heat olive oil over medium heat.
2. Add mushrooms, onion, and garlic. Sauté until tender.
3. Add bone broth and bring to a simmer.
4. In a small bowl, dissolve arrowroot powder in a little water and add to the saucepan.
5. Stir until the gravy thickens.
6. Season with coconut aminos, salt, and pepper to taste.
7. Store in the refrigerator for up to one week.

Health Problems Addressed: Inflammation

Health Benefits: High in antioxidants and nutrients

Scientific Benefits: Mushrooms provide antioxidants and bone broth supports gut health

"This gravy is savory and rich, perfect for meats and mashed vegetables."

275. Sweet Potato Hummus

Ingredients:
- 1 large sweet potato, roasted and peeled
- 1/4 cup tahini
- 2 tablespoons lemon juice
- 1 clove garlic, minced
- 1/4 cup olive oil
- Salt and pepper to taste

Instructions:
1. In a blender, combine roasted sweet potato, tahini, lemon juice, garlic, and olive oil.
2. Blend until smooth.
3. Season with salt and pepper to taste.
4. Store in the refrigerator for up to one week.

Health Problems Addressed: Inflammation, nutrient deficiencies

Health Benefits: High in vitamins and antioxidants

Scientific Benefits: Sweet potatoes provide vitamins A and C, and tahini offers healthy fats and protein

"This hummus is sweet and creamy, perfect for dipping vegetables or spreading on crackers."

276. Lemon Poppy Seed Dressing

Ingredients:
- 1/4 cup olive oil
- 2 tablespoons fresh lemon juice
- 1 tablespoon honey or maple syrup
- 1 teaspoon Dijon mustard (AIP compliant)
- 1 teaspoon poppy seeds
- Salt and pepper to taste

Instructions:
1. In a bowl, whisk together olive oil, lemon juice, honey or maple syrup, Dijon mustard, and poppy seeds.
2. Season with salt and pepper to taste.
3. Store in the refrigerator for up to one week.

Health Problems Addressed: Inflammation

Health Benefits: High in healthy fats and antioxidants

Scientific Benefits: Olive oil provides healthy fats, and lemon juice has vitamin C and antioxidant properties

"This dressing is tangy and sweet, perfect for salads and as a marinade."

277. Roasted Red Pepper Pesto

Ingredients:
- 2 roasted red bell peppers, peeled and seeded
- 1/4 cup olive oil
- 1/4 cup fresh basil leaves
- 2 cloves garlic, minced
- 1 tablespoon nutritional yeast (optional)
- Salt and pepper to taste

Instructions:
1. In a blender, combine roasted red bell peppers, olive oil, basil, garlic, and nutritional yeast (if using).
2. Blend until smooth.
3. Season with salt and pepper to taste.
4. Store in the refrigerator for up to one week.

Health Problems Addressed: Inflammation

Health Benefits: High in vitamins and antioxidants

Scientific Benefits: Red bell peppers provide vitamins and antioxidants, and basil has anti-inflammatory properties

"This pesto is vibrant and flavorful, perfect for pasta or as a spread."

278. Ginger Carrot Dressing

Ingredients:
- 1/2 cup carrot juice
- 1 tablespoon fresh ginger, grated
- 2 tablespoons olive oil
- 1 tablespoon apple cider vinegar
- 1 clove garlic, minced
- Salt and pepper to taste

Instructions:
1. In a bowl, whisk together carrot juice, ginger, olive oil, apple cider vinegar, and garlic.
2. Season with salt and pepper to taste.
3. Store in the refrigerator for up to one week.

Health Problems Addressed: Inflammation, digestive issues

Health Benefits: High in vitamins and antioxidants

Scientific Benefits: Carrot juice provides vitamins and antioxidants, and ginger has anti-inflammatory and digestive properties

"This dressing is tangy and refreshing, perfect for salads and as a marinade."

279. Cilantro Lime Sauce

Ingredients:
- 1 cup fresh cilantro leaves
- 1/4 cup olive oil
- 2 tablespoons lime juice
- 1 clove garlic, minced
- Salt to taste

Instructions:
1. In a blender, combine cilantro, olive oil, lime juice, and garlic.
2. Blend until smooth.
3. Season with salt to taste.
4. Store in the refrigerator for up to one week.

Health Problems Addressed: Inflammation

Health Benefits: High in vitamins and antioxidants

Scientific Benefits: Cilantro provides vitamins and antioxidants, and lime juice has vitamin C and antioxidant properties

"This sauce is fresh and zesty, perfect for drizzling over tacos and grilled meats."

280. Apple Cider Vinaigrette

Ingredients:
- 1/4 cup apple cider vinegar
- 1/4 cup olive oil
- 1 tablespoon honey or maple syrup
- 1 teaspoon Dijon mustard (AIP compliant)
- Salt and pepper to taste

Instructions:
1. In a bowl, whisk together apple cider vinegar, olive oil, honey or maple syrup, and Dijon mustard.
2. Season with salt and pepper to taste.
3. Store in the refrigerator for up to one week.

Health Problems Addressed: Inflammation

Health Benefits: High in antioxidants and healthy fats

Scientific Benefits: Apple cider vinegar has anti-inflammatory properties, and olive oil provides healthy fats

"This vinaigrette is tangy and sweet, perfect for salads and as a marinade."

281. Spiced Pumpkin Dip

Ingredients:
- 1 cup pumpkin puree
- 1/4 cup tahini
- 2 tablespoons maple syrup
- 1 teaspoon ground cinnamon
- 1/2 teaspoon ground ginger
- Salt to taste

Instructions:
1. In a bowl, combine pumpkin puree, tahini, maple syrup, cinnamon, and ginger.
2. Mix well.
3. Season with salt to taste.
4. Store in the refrigerator for up to one week.

Health Problems Addressed: Inflammation, nutrient deficiencies

Health Benefits: High in vitamins and antioxidants

Scientific Benefits: Pumpkin provides vitamins A and C, and tahini offers healthy fats and protein

"This dip is creamy and spiced, perfect for dipping fruits and spreading on crackers."

282. Basil Pesto

Ingredients:
- 1 cup fresh basil leaves
- 1/4 cup olive oil
- 2 cloves garlic, minced
- 1/4 cup pine nuts (optional)
- Salt and pepper to taste

Instructions:
1. In a blender, combine basil leaves, olive oil, garlic, and pine nuts (if using).
2. Blend until smooth.
3. Season with salt and pepper to taste.
4. Store in the refrigerator for up to one week.

Health Problems Addressed: Inflammation

Health Benefits: High in vitamins and healthy fats

Scientific Benefits: Basil provides anti-inflammatory properties, and olive oil offers healthy fats

"This pesto is fresh and aromatic, perfect for pasta, sandwiches, and as a dip."

283. Avocado Lime Crema

Ingredients:
- 1 ripe avocado
- 2 tablespoons lime juice
- 1/4 cup coconut yogurt (AIP compliant)
- 1 clove garlic, minced
- Salt to taste

Instructions:
1. In a blender, combine avocado, lime juice, coconut yogurt, and garlic.
2. Blend until smooth.
3. Season with salt to taste.
4. Store in the refrigerator for up to three days.

Health Problems Addressed: Inflammation, nutrient deficiencies

Health Benefits: High in healthy fats and vitamins

Scientific Benefits: Avocado provides healthy fats and vitamins, and lime juice has antioxidant properties

"This crema is creamy and tangy, perfect for topping tacos and grilled vegetables."

284. Mustard Dill Sauce

Ingredients:
- 1/4 cup Dijon mustard (AIP compliant)
- 2 tablespoons fresh dill, chopped
- 1 tablespoon honey or maple syrup
- 1 tablespoon apple cider vinegar
- Salt and pepper to taste

Instructions:
1. In a bowl, whisk together Dijon mustard, dill, honey or maple syrup, and apple cider vinegar.
2. Season with salt and pepper to taste.
3. Store in the refrigerator for up to one week.

Health Problems Addressed: Inflammation

Health Benefits: High in antioxidants and vitamins

Scientific Benefits: Dill has antioxidant properties, and apple cider vinegar is anti-inflammatory

"This sauce is tangy and herby, perfect for salmon and roasted vegetables."

285. Roasted Tomato Salsa

Ingredients:
- 4 medium tomatoes, roasted and chopped
- 1/4 cup red onion, finely chopped
- 2 tablespoons fresh cilantro, chopped
- 1 jalapeño, seeded and finely chopped
- 2 tablespoons lime juice
- Salt to taste

Instructions:
1. In a bowl, combine roasted tomatoes, red onion, cilantro, jalapeño, and lime juice.
2. Mix well.
3. Season with salt to taste.
4. Store in the refrigerator for up to three days.

Health Problems Addressed: Inflammation

Health Benefits: High in vitamins and antioxidants

Scientific Benefits: Tomatoes provide vitamins and antioxidants, and lime juice has vitamin C

"This salsa is smoky and fresh, perfect for dipping and topping grilled meats."

286. Coconut Mint Chutney

Ingredients:
- 1 cup fresh mint leaves
- 1/4 cup shredded coconut
- 2 tablespoons lime juice
- 1 clove garlic, minced
- 1 tablespoon honey or maple syrup
- Salt to taste

Instructions:
1. In a blender, combine mint leaves, shredded coconut, lime juice, garlic, and honey or maple syrup.
2. Blend until smooth.
3. Season with salt to taste.
4. Store in the refrigerator for up to one week.

Health Problems Addressed: Inflammation, digestive issues

Health Benefits: High in vitamins and antioxidants

Scientific Benefits: Mint provides antioxidants and aids digestion, and coconut offers healthy fats

"This chutney is refreshing and sweet, perfect for adding a burst of flavor to dishes."

287. Lemon Dill Aioli

Ingredients:
- 1/2 cup mayonnaise (AIP compliant)
- 1 tablespoon fresh lemon juice
- 1 tablespoon fresh dill, chopped
- 1 clove garlic, minced
- Salt and pepper to taste

Instructions:
1. In a bowl, whisk together mayonnaise, lemon juice, dill, and garlic.
2. Season with salt and pepper to taste.
3. Store in the refrigerator for up to one week.

Health Problems Addressed: Inflammation

Health Benefits: High in healthy fats

Scientific Benefits: Dill and lemon juice provide antioxidants and anti-inflammatory properties

"This aioli is creamy and tangy, perfect for dipping and spreading."

288. Green Olive Tapenade

Ingredients:
- 1 cup green olives, pitted and chopped
- 1/4 cup olive oil
- 1 clove garlic, minced
- 2 tablespoons fresh parsley, chopped
- 1 tablespoon capers, rinsed
- Salt and pepper to taste

Instructions:
1. In a bowl, combine green olives, olive oil, garlic, parsley, and capers.
2. Mix well.
3. Season with salt and pepper to taste.
4. Store in the refrigerator for up to one week.

Health Problems Addressed: Inflammation

Health Benefits: High in healthy fats and antioxidants

Scientific Benefits: Olives provide healthy fats and antioxidants

"This tapenade is savory and briny, perfect for spreading on crackers or as a dip."

289. Spicy Mango Chutney

Ingredients:
- 1 ripe mango, peeled and diced
- 1/4 cup red onion, finely chopped
- 1 jalapeño, seeded and finely chopped
- 2 tablespoons lime juice
- 1 tablespoon honey or maple syrup
- Salt to taste

Instructions:
1. In a bowl, combine mango, red onion, jalapeño, lime juice, and honey or maple syrup.
2. Mix well.
3. Season with salt to taste.
4. Store in the refrigerator for up to three days.

Health Problems Addressed: Inflammation

Health Benefits: High in vitamins and antioxidants

Scientific Benefits: Mango provides vitamins and antioxidants, and jalapeño has anti-inflammatory properties

"This chutney is sweet and spicy, perfect for adding a kick to dishes."

290. Sun-Dried Tomato Tapenade

Ingredients:
- 1/2 cup sun-dried tomatoes (not in oil), soaked and chopped
- 1/4 cup olive oil
- 2 tablespoons fresh basil, chopped
- 1 clove garlic, minced
- 1 tablespoon capers, rinsed
- Salt and pepper to taste

Instructions:
1. In a bowl, combine sun-dried tomatoes, olive oil, basil, garlic, and capers.
2. Mix well.
3. Season with salt and pepper to taste.
4. Store in the refrigerator for up to one week.

Health Problems Addressed: Inflammation

Health Benefits: High in vitamins and antioxidants

Scientific Benefits: Sun-dried tomatoes provide vitamins and antioxidants

"This tapenade is rich and flavorful, perfect for spreading on bread or as a dip."

291. Carrot Ginger Soup

Ingredients:
- 4 large carrots, peeled and chopped
- 1 onion, chopped
- 2 cloves garlic, minced
- 1 tablespoon fresh ginger, grated
- 4 cups bone broth
- 2 tablespoons coconut cream
- Salt and pepper to taste

Instructions:
1. In a pot, sauté onions, garlic, and ginger until fragrant.
2. Add carrots and bone broth.
3. Simmer until carrots are tender.
4. Blend until smooth.
5. Stir in coconut cream.
6. Season with salt and pepper to taste.

Health Problems Addressed: Inflammation, digestive issues

Health Benefits: High in vitamins and antioxidants

Scientific Benefits: Carrots provide vitamins and antioxidants, and ginger aids digestion

"This soup is creamy and warming, perfect for a comforting meal."

292. Creamy Beet Soup

Ingredients:
- 4 medium beets, roasted and peeled
- 1 onion, chopped
- 2 cloves garlic, minced
- 4 cups bone broth
- 2 tablespoons coconut cream
- Salt and pepper to taste

Instructions:
1. In a pot, sauté onions and garlic until fragrant.
2. Add roasted beets and bone broth.
3. Simmer until the beets are tender.
4. Blend until smooth.
5. Stir in coconut cream.
6. Season with salt and pepper to taste.

Health Problems Addressed: Inflammation, nutrient deficiencies

Health Benefits: High in vitamins and antioxidants

Scientific Benefits: Beets provide antioxidants and nutrients

"This soup is vibrant and creamy, perfect for a nourishing meal."

293. Cauliflower Alfredo Sauce

Ingredients:
- 1 head cauliflower, chopped
- 2 cloves garlic, minced
- 1 cup bone broth
- 1/4 cup nutritional yeast (optional)
- 1/4 cup coconut cream
- Salt and pepper to taste

Instructions:
1. In a pot, simmer cauliflower and garlic in bone broth until tender.
2. Blend until smooth.
3. Stir in nutritional yeast (if using) and coconut cream.
4. Season with salt and pepper to taste.

Health Problems Addressed: Inflammation, digestive issues

Health Benefits: High in vitamins and nutrients

Scientific Benefits: Cauliflower provides vitamins and antioxidants

"This Alfredo sauce is creamy and delicious, perfect for pasta and vegetables."

294. Basil Lemon Vinaigrette

Ingredients:
- 1/4 cup olive oil
- 2 tablespoons fresh lemon juice
- 1/4 cup fresh basil leaves, chopped
- 1 clove garlic, minced
- Salt and pepper to taste

Instructions:
1. In a bowl, whisk together olive oil, lemon juice, basil, and garlic.
2. Season with salt and pepper to taste.
3. Store in the refrigerator for up to one week.

Health Problems Addressed: Inflammation

Health Benefits: High in antioxidants and healthy fats

Scientific Benefits: Basil provides anti-inflammatory properties, and olive oil offers healthy fats

"This vinaigrette is fresh and tangy, perfect for salads and as a marinade."

295. Sweet Potato Tahini Sauce

Ingredients:
- 1 large sweet potato, roasted and peeled
- 1/4 cup tahini
- 2 tablespoons lemon juice
- 1 clove garlic, minced
- 1/4 cup olive oil
- Salt and pepper to taste

Instructions:
1. In a blender, combine roasted sweet potato, tahini, lemon juice, garlic, and olive oil.
2. Blend until smooth.
3. Season with salt and pepper to taste.
4. Store in the refrigerator for up to one week.

Health Problems Addressed: Inflammation, nutrient deficiencies

Health Benefits: High in vitamins and antioxidants

Scientific Benefits: Sweet potatoes provide vitamins A and C, and tahini offers healthy fats and protein

"This sauce is creamy and nutty, perfect for dipping and spreading."

296. Coconut Milk Ranch Dressing

Ingredients:
- 1/2 cup coconut milk
- 2 tablespoons fresh dill, chopped
- 2 tablespoons fresh chives, chopped
- 1 tablespoon fresh parsley, chopped
- 1 tablespoon apple cider vinegar
- 1 clove garlic, minced
- Salt and pepper to taste

Instructions:
1. In a bowl, whisk together coconut milk, dill, chives, parsley, apple cider vinegar, and garlic.
2. Season with salt and pepper to taste.
3. Store in the refrigerator for up to one week.

Health Problems Addressed: Inflammation

Health Benefits: High in healthy fats and vitamins

Scientific Benefits: Coconut milk provides healthy fats, and herbs offer antioxidant properties

"This ranch dressing is creamy and herby, perfect for salads and dipping."

297. Spicy Avocado Salsa

Ingredients:
- 2 ripe avocados, diced
- 1/4 cup red onion, finely chopped
- 1 jalapeño, seeded and finely chopped
- 2 tablespoons lime juice
- 2 tablespoons fresh cilantro, chopped
- Salt to taste

Instructions:
1. In a bowl, combine avocados, red onion, jalapeño, lime juice, and cilantro.
2. Mix well.
3. Season with salt to taste.
4. Store in the refrigerator for up to three days.

Health Problems Addressed: Inflammation

Health Benefits: High in healthy fats and vitamins

Scientific Benefits: Avocado provides healthy fats and vitamins, and jalapeño has anti-inflammatory properties

"This salsa is creamy and spicy, perfect for topping tacos and grilled meats."

298. Almond Butter Sauce

Ingredients:
- 1/4 cup almond butter
- 2 tablespoons coconut aminos
- 1 tablespoon fresh lime juice
- 1 tablespoon honey or maple syrup
- 1 clove garlic, minced
- 1/4 cup water (as needed)
- Salt to taste

Instructions:
1. In a bowl, whisk together almond butter, coconut aminos, lime juice, honey or maple syrup, and garlic.
2. Add water to reach desired consistency.
3. Season with salt to taste.
4. Store in the refrigerator for up to one week.

Health Problems Addressed: Inflammation

Health Benefits: High in healthy fats and protein

Scientific Benefits: Almond butter provides healthy fats and protein

"This sauce is creamy and nutty, perfect for drizzling over vegetables and meats."

299. Lemon Garlic Tahini Sauce

Ingredients:
- 1/4 cup tahini
- 2 tablespoons fresh lemon juice
- 1 clove garlic, minced
- 2 tablespoons water (as needed)
- Salt to taste

Instructions:
1. In a bowl, whisk together tahini, lemon juice, and garlic.
2. Add water to reach desired consistency.
3. Season with salt to taste.
4. Store in the refrigerator for up to one week.

Health Problems Addressed: Inflammation

Health Benefits: High in healthy fats and vitamins

Scientific Benefits: Tahini provides healthy fats and protein, and lemon juice offers antioxidant properties

"This sauce is tangy and nutty, perfect for drizzling over salads and roasted vegetables."

300. Cilantro Lime Yogurt Sauce

Ingredients:
- 1/2 cup coconut yogurt (AIP compliant)

- 1/4 cup fresh cilantro, chopped
- 2 tablespoons lime juice
- 1 clove garlic, minced
- Salt to taste

Instructions:
1. In a bowl, whisk together coconut yogurt, cilantro, lime juice, and garlic.
2. Season with salt to taste.
3. Store in the refrigerator for up to one week.

Health Problems Addressed: Inflammation, digestive issues

Health Benefits: High in probiotics and vitamins

Scientific Benefits: Coconut yogurt provides probiotics, and cilantro offers antioxidants

"This sauce is creamy and fresh, perfect for topping tacos and grilled vegetables."

Chapter 8: Meal Plans

7-Day Meal Plan for Beginners

Day 1

Breakfast: Sweet Potato Hash with Spinach and Sausage (Recipe 1)

Lunch: Grilled Chicken Salad with Mango Salsa (Recipe 56)

Dinner: Lemon Herb Salmon with Asparagus (Recipe 116)

Snack: Apple Slices with Cinnamon Coconut Butter (Recipe 162)

Day 2

Breakfast: Blueberry Coconut Smoothie (Recipe 6)

Lunch: Turkey and Avocado Lettuce Wraps (Recipe 68)

Dinner: Beef and Broccoli Stir-Fry (Recipe 131)

Snack: Plantain Chips with Guacamole (Recipe 155)

Day 3

Breakfast: Carrot Cake Porridge (Recipe 7)

Lunch: Butternut Squash Soup (Recipe 75)

Dinner: Balsamic Chicken with Roasted Vegetables (Recipe 138)

Snack: Kale Chips (Recipe 172)

Day 4

Breakfast: Green Smoothie Bowl (Recipe 8)
Lunch: Zucchini Noodles with Pesto (Recipe 79)
Dinner: Lamb Chops with Mint Sauce (Recipe 145)
Snack: Cucumber Hummus Bites (Recipe 178)

Day 5

Breakfast: Pumpkin Spice Latte (Recipe 9)
Lunch: Grilled Shrimp Salad (Recipe 86)
Dinner: Pork Tenderloin with Apple Compote (Recipe 147)
Snack: Coconut Energy Balls (Recipe 181)

Day 6

Breakfast: Strawberry Chia Pudding (Recipe 10)
Lunch: Cauliflower Rice Sushi Bowls (Recipe 89)
Dinner: Chicken Alfredo with Zoodles (Recipe 149)
Snack: Seaweed Snacks (Recipe 183)

Day 7

Breakfast: Banana Pancakes with Blueberry Sauce (Recipe 11)
Lunch: Chicken Caesar Salad (Recipe 91)
Dinner: Braised Short Ribs with Mashed Cauliflower (Recipe 150)
Snack: Apple Chips (Recipe 185)

30-Day Autoimmune Paleo Diet Reset Plan

This 30-Day Reset Plan is designed to help you transition into the Autoimmune Paleo (AIP) diet smoothly, eliminate potential triggers of inflammation, and promote healing. This plan includes a variety of delicious recipes for breakfasts, lunches, dinners, and snacks, along with tips to stay on track.

Week 1

Day 1
Breakfast: Sweet Potato Hash with Spinach and Sausage (Recipe 1)
Lunch: Grilled Chicken Salad with Mango Salsa (Recipe 56)
Dinner: Lemon Herb Salmon with Asparagus (Recipe 116)
Snack: Apple Slices with Cinnamon Coconut Butter (Recipe 162)

Day 2
Breakfast: Blueberry Coconut Smoothie (Recipe 6)
Lunch: Turkey and Avocado Lettuce Wraps (Recipe 68)
Dinner: Beef and Broccoli Stir-Fry (Recipe 131)
Snack: Plantain Chips with Guacamole (Recipe 155)

Day 3

Breakfast: Carrot Cake Porridge (Recipe 7)

Lunch: Butternut Squash Soup (Recipe 75)

Dinner: Balsamic Chicken with Roasted Vegetables (Recipe 138)

Snack: Kale Chips (Recipe 172)

Day 4

Breakfast: Green Smoothie Bowl (Recipe 8)

Lunch: Zucchini Noodles with Pesto (Recipe 79)

Dinner: Lamb Chops with Mint Sauce (Recipe 145)

Snack: Cucumber Hummus Bites (Recipe 178)

Day 5

Breakfast: Pumpkin Spice Latte (Recipe 9)

Lunch: Grilled Shrimp Salad (Recipe 86)

Dinner: Pork Tenderloin with Apple Compote (Recipe 147)

Snack: Coconut Energy Balls (Recipe 181)

Day 6

Breakfast: Strawberry Chia Pudding (Recipe 10)

Lunch: Cauliflower Rice Sushi Bowls (Recipe 89)

Dinner: Chicken Alfredo with Zoodles (Recipe 149)

Snack: Seaweed Snacks (Recipe 183)

Day 7

Breakfast: Banana Pancakes with Blueberry Sauce (Recipe 11)
Lunch: Chicken Caesar Salad (Recipe 91)
Dinner: Braised Short Ribs with Mashed Cauliflower (Recipe 150)
Snack: Apple Chips (Recipe 185)

Week 2

Day 8
Breakfast: Sweet Potato Hash with Spinach and Sausage (Recipe 1)
Lunch: Grilled Chicken Salad with Mango Salsa (Recipe 56)
Dinner: Lemon Herb Salmon with Asparagus (Recipe 116)
Snack: Apple Slices with Cinnamon Coconut Butter (Recipe 162)

Day 9
Breakfast: Blueberry Coconut Smoothie (Recipe 6)
Lunch: Turkey and Avocado Lettuce Wraps (Recipe 68)
Dinner: Beef and Broccoli Stir-Fry (Recipe 131)
Snack: Plantain Chips with Guacamole (Recipe 155)

Day 10
Breakfast: Carrot Cake Porridge (Recipe 7)
Lunch: Butternut Squash Soup (Recipe 75)

Dinner: Balsamic Chicken with Roasted Vegetables (Recipe 138)
Snack: Kale Chips (Recipe 172)

Day 11
Breakfast: Green Smoothie Bowl (Recipe 8)
Lunch: Zucchini Noodles with Pesto (Recipe 79)
Dinner: Lamb Chops with Mint Sauce (Recipe 145)
Snack: Cucumber Hummus Bites (Recipe 178)

Day 12
Breakfast: Pumpkin Spice Latte (Recipe 9)
Lunch: Grilled Shrimp Salad (Recipe 86)
Dinner: Pork Tenderloin with Apple Compote (Recipe 147)
Snack: Coconut Energy Balls (Recipe 181)

Day 13
Breakfast: Strawberry Chia Pudding (Recipe 10)
Lunch: Cauliflower Rice Sushi Bowls (Recipe 89)
Dinner: Chicken Alfredo with Zoodles (Recipe 149)
Snack: Seaweed Snacks (Recipe 183)

Day 14
Breakfast: Banana Pancakes with Blueberry Sauce (Recipe 11)
Lunch: Chicken Caesar Salad (Recipe 91)

Dinner: Braised Short Ribs with Mashed Cauliflower
(Recipe 150)
Snack: Apple Chips (Recipe 185)

Week 3

Day 15

Breakfast: Sweet Potato Hash with Spinach and Sausage
(Recipe 1)
Lunch: Grilled Chicken Salad with Mango Salsa (Recipe
56)
Dinner: Lemon Herb Salmon with Asparagus (Recipe
116)
Snack: Apple Slices with Cinnamon Coconut Butter
(Recipe 162)

Day 16

Breakfast: Blueberry Coconut Smoothie (Recipe 6)
Lunch: Turkey and Avocado Lettuce Wraps (Recipe 68)
Dinner: Beef and Broccoli Stir-Fry (Recipe 131)
Snack: Plantain Chips with Guacamole (Recipe 155)

Day 17

Breakfast: Carrot Cake Porridge (Recipe 7)
Lunch: Butternut Squash Soup (Recipe 75)
Dinner: Balsamic Chicken with Roasted Vegetables
(Recipe 138)
Snack: Kale Chips (Recipe 172)

Day 18
Breakfast: Green Smoothie Bowl (Recipe 8)
Lunch: Zucchini Noodles with Pesto (Recipe 79)
Dinner: Lamb Chops with Mint Sauce (Recipe 145)
Snack: Cucumber Hummus Bites (Recipe 178)

Day 19
Breakfast: Pumpkin Spice Latte (Recipe 9)
Lunch: Grilled Shrimp Salad (Recipe 86)
Dinner: Pork Tenderloin with Apple Compote (Recipe 147)
Snack: Coconut Energy Balls (Recipe 181)

Day 20
Breakfast: Strawberry Chia Pudding (Recipe 10)
Lunch: Cauliflower Rice Sushi Bowls (Recipe 89)
Dinner: Chicken Alfredo with Zoodles (Recipe 149)
Snack: Seaweed Snacks (Recipe 183)

Day 21
Breakfast: Banana Pancakes with Blueberry Sauce (Recipe 11)
Lunch: Chicken Caesar Salad (Recipe 91)
Dinner: Braised Short Ribs with Mashed Cauliflower (Recipe 150)
Snack: Apple Chips (Recipe 185)

Week 4

Day 22
Breakfast: Sweet Potato Hash with Spinach and Sausage (Recipe 1)
Lunch: Grilled Chicken Salad with Mango Salsa (Recipe 56)
Dinner: Lemon Herb Salmon with Asparagus (Recipe 116)
Snack: Apple Slices with Cinnamon Coconut Butter (Recipe 162)

Day 23
Breakfast: Blueberry Coconut Smoothie (Recipe 6)
Lunch: Turkey and Avocado Lettuce Wraps (Recipe 68)
Dinner: Beef and Broccoli Stir-Fry (Recipe 131)
Snack: Plantain Chips with Guacamole (Recipe 155)

Day 24
Breakfast: Carrot Cake Porridge (Recipe 7)
Lunch: Butternut Squash Soup (Recipe 75)
Dinner: Balsamic Chicken with Roasted Vegetables (Recipe 138)
Snack: Kale Chips (Recipe 172)

Day 25
Breakfast: Green Smoothie Bowl (Recipe 8)
Lunch: Zucchini Noodles with Pesto (Recipe 79)

Dinner: Lamb Chops with Mint Sauce (Recipe 145)
Snack: Cucumber Hummus Bites (Recipe 178)

Day 26

Breakfast: Pumpkin Spice Latte (Recipe 9)
Lunch: Grilled Shrimp Salad (Recipe 86)
Dinner: Pork Tenderloin with Apple Compote (Recipe 147)
Snack: Coconut Energy Balls (Recipe 181)

Day 27

Breakfast: Strawberry Chia Pudding (Recipe 10)
Lunch: Cauliflower Rice Sushi Bowls (Recipe 89)
Dinner: Chicken Alfredo with Zoodles (Recipe 149)
Snack: Seaweed Snacks (Recipe 183)

Day 28

Breakfast: Banana Pancakes with Blueberry Sauce (Recipe 11)
Lunch: Chicken Caesar Salad (Recipe 91)
Dinner: Braised Short Ribs with Mashed Cauliflower (Recipe 150)
Snack: Apple Chips (Recipe 185)

Day 29

Breakfast: Sweet Potato Hash with Spinach and Sausage (Recipe 1)

Lunch: Grilled Chicken Salad with Mango Salsa (Recipe 56)

Dinner: Lemon Herb Salmon with Asparagus (Recipe 116)

Snack: Apple Slices with Cinnamon Coconut Butter (Recipe 162)

Day 30

Breakfast: Blueberry Coconut Smoothie (Recipe 6)

Lunch: Turkey and Avocado Lettuce Wraps (Recipe 68)

Dinner: Beef and Broccoli Stir-Fry (Recipe 131)

Snack: Plantain Chips with Guacamole (Recipe 155)

Tips to Stay on Track

1. Meal Prep: Spend a few hours each week preparing meals and snacks in advance.

2. Variety: Rotate recipes and try new ones to keep meals exciting.

3. Support: Join AIP communities online for support and recipe ideas.

4. Listen to Your Body: Pay attention to how foods make you feel and adjust your diet accordingly.

5. Stay Hydrated: Drink plenty of water throughout the day.

The 30-Day Reset Plan is a comprehensive guide to help you start and stick with the AIP diet. By following this plan, you can eliminate potential triggers, reduce inflammation, and support your body's natural healing process. Remember, the journey to health is unique for everyone, so be patient with yourself and enjoy the delicious, nourishing foods that the AIP diet offers.

Conclusion

Maintaining a Healthy Lifestyle

Embarking on the Autoimmune Paleo (AIP) diet journey is a powerful step towards managing autoimmune conditions and promoting overall health. However, maintaining this lifestyle can be challenging. Here are some tips to help you continue with the AIP diet and make sustainable, healthy lifestyle changes:

1. Stay Informed and Educated
- Continuously educate yourself about autoimmune conditions and the benefits of the AIP diet. Knowledge empowers you to make informed decisions about your health and diet.

2. Plan Ahead
- Consistently plan your meals and snacks. This ensures that you always have AIP-compliant options available, reducing the temptation to stray from the diet.

3. Keep a Food Journal
- Track what you eat and how it makes you feel. This helps identify any foods that may trigger symptoms and allows you to fine-tune your diet for optimal health.

4. Embrace Variety

- Experiment with new recipes and ingredients. A diverse diet not only ensures a broad range of nutrients but also keeps meals interesting and enjoyable.

5. Batch Cooking and Meal Prep

- Set aside time each week for batch cooking and meal prep. Having ready-to-eat meals and snacks saves time and makes it easier to stick to your diet.

6. Find Support

- Connect with others who are following the AIP diet. Join online communities, local support groups, or find a buddy to share recipes, tips, and encouragement.

7. Listen to Your Body

- Pay attention to how your body responds to different foods and lifestyle changes. Personalize the diet to fit your unique needs and preferences.

8. Practice Self-Care

- Manage stress through practices like meditation, yoga, or gentle exercise. Prioritize sleep and engage in activities that promote mental and emotional well-being.

9. Celebrate Small Wins

- Recognize and celebrate your progress, no matter how small. Acknowledge improvements in your health and well-being as motivation to continue.

10. Be Flexible and Patient
- Understand that everyone's journey is different. Be patient with yourself and flexible in your approach. It's okay to make adjustments as needed.

Sustainable Lifestyle Changes

1. Balanced Nutrition
- Aim for a balanced intake of proteins, fats, and carbohydrates. Focus on whole, nutrient-dense foods that support overall health.

2. Regular Physical Activity
- Incorporate regular exercise that you enjoy. Physical activity enhances mood, supports immune function, and improves overall health.

3. Mindful Eating
- Practice mindful eating by savoring each bite and paying attention to hunger and fullness cues. This can prevent overeating and improve digestion.

4. Hydration

- Stay hydrated by drinking plenty of water throughout the day. Proper hydration supports all bodily functions and enhances overall health.

5. Continuous Learning
- Stay curious and open to learning about new foods, recipes, and health strategies. Continual learning helps keep your diet and lifestyle fresh and exciting.

6. Holistic Approach
- Consider a holistic approach to health that includes not only diet but also physical activity, stress management, and emotional well-being.

By integrating these tips and strategies into your daily routine, you can maintain a healthy, sustainable lifestyle that supports your journey on the AIP diet. Remember, the goal is to feel better, manage symptoms, and improve your overall quality of life. Your commitment to your health is commendable, and every step you take brings you closer to optimal wellness.

Thank you for choosing this cookbook as a guide on your journey to health and wellness. The recipes, meal plans, and tips provided are designed to support you in managing your autoimmune condition and enjoying a fulfilling, delicious diet. As you continue to explore the world of AIP-friendly foods, may you find joy,

nourishment, and a renewed sense of well-being. Here's
to your health and happiness!